Chapter 1: Understanding Parkinson's Disease

Overview of Parkinson's Disease

Parkinson's Disease is a progressive neurodegenerative disorder that primarily affects movement. It occurs when certain nerve cells, or neurons, in the brain gradually break down or die. This leads to a decrease in dopamine production, a neurotransmitter that plays a crucial role in sending messages to the part of the brain that controls movement and coordination. The exact cause of Parkinson's disease remains unclear, although a combination of genetic and environmental factors is believed to contribute to its development. Understanding the basic mechanisms of this disease is essential for patients and caregivers alike as they navigate its early signs and impacts on daily life.

The early symptoms of Parkinson's disease can be subtle and may vary significantly from person to person. Common early signs include tremors, stiffness, slowness of movement, and balance problems. Many patients also experience changes in their handwriting, known as micrographia, and may notice a decrease in their sense of smell. These early indicators can often be mistaken for normal aging or other conditions, which underscores the importance of awareness and education regarding the disease. Recognizing these signs early can lead to timely diagnosis and intervention, ultimately improving quality of life.

Nutrition and diet play a pivotal role in managing Parkinson's disease. Research suggests that a balanced diet rich in antioxidants, omega-3 fatty acids, and fiber can help alleviate some symptoms and promote overall health. Certain nutrients may also support brain health and potentially slow disease progression. Patients are encouraged to work with healthcare professionals to develop personalized meal plans that meet their specific nutritional needs. Additionally, staying hydrated and maintaining a healthy weight are important considerations for managing the disease effectively.

Exercise and physical therapy are vital components of a comprehensive management plan for Parkinson's disease. Regular physical activity helps improve mobility, flexibility, and balance, which can counteract some of the physical limitations caused by the disease. Tailored exercise programs, including strength training, aerobic activity, and stretching, can enhance physical function and reduce the risk of falls. Furthermore, engaging in activities such as dancing or tai chi can be particularly beneficial, as they not only promote physical health but also provide social interaction and enjoyment.

Finally, understanding the emotional and psychological aspects of living with Parkinson's disease is crucial. Many patients and caregivers experience feelings of anxiety, depression, or isolation as they cope with the challenges posed by the disease. Community support groups can offer valuable resources and a sense of connection among individuals facing similar struggles. Moreover, advances in research are continually uncovering new treatment options and alternative therapies, providing hope for improved management of the disease. By fostering a strong support network and staying informed about the latest developments in Parkinson's research, patients and caregivers can navigate their journey with greater confidence and resilience.

Early Signs and Symptoms

Recognizing the early signs and symptoms of Parkinson's disease is crucial for timely diagnosis and intervention. Many individuals may overlook subtle changes in their bodies, attributing them to aging or stress. However, understanding these early indicators can empower patients and caregivers alike to seek medical advice sooner rather than later. Common early symptoms include tremors, stiffness, and changes in balance. These manifestations can significantly impact daily activities and quality of life, making awareness an essential component of managing Parkinson's effectively.

Tremors are often one of the first signs that individuals notice. These tremors typically begin in one hand or foot and may appear as a slight shaking or trembling. While hand tremors are commonly associated with Parkinson's, they can also manifest in other parts of the body, such as the jaw or leg. It is important to distinguish these tremors from other causes, as not all shaking is indicative of Parkinson's disease. Patients should monitor the frequency and severity of tremors and discuss them with healthcare professionals to determine the best course of action.

Another early symptom is rigidity or stiffness in the muscles. This can lead to discomfort and can affect mobility. Patients may experience difficulty in initiating movements, which can be particularly concerning when it affects simple tasks such as getting out of a chair or walking. As stiffness progresses, it may also impact posture and overall balance. Recognizing these changes early can help patients engage in appropriate physical therapy and exercise routines that promote flexibility and strength, which are crucial for maintaining mobility and independence.

Changes in facial expressions, often referred to as "masked face," can also be an early indication of Parkinson's disease. Individuals may notice a reduction in spontaneous facial movements, resulting in a less expressive appearance. This can affect social interactions and communication, leading to misunderstandings with family and friends. Being aware of these changes can facilitate discussions with caregivers and loved ones, creating a supportive environment that addresses emotional and mental health concerns.

Lastly, early signs can encompass changes in sleep patterns and cognitive function. Many patients report difficulties with sleep, including insomnia or restless leg syndrome, which can exacerbate fatigue and affect overall well-being. Cognitive changes such as difficulties with concentration or memory may also occur. Engaging in community support groups or seeking mental health resources can provide valuable tools for coping with these symptoms. Understanding and recognizing these early signs not only aids in seeking timely medical intervention but also reinforces the importance of a comprehensive approach to managing Parkinson's disease through nutrition, exercise, and support systems.

Importance of Early Detection

Early detection of Parkinson's disease is crucial in managing the condition effectively and improving the overall quality of life for patients. Recognizing the early symptoms can lead to timely interventions that may slow the progression of the disease. Symptoms such as subtle changes in movement, tremors, or even shifts in emotional well-being can be easily overlooked or attributed to aging. However, being vigilant about these signs can facilitate earlier diagnosis and the initiation of treatment plans tailored to individual needs.

Receiving a diagnosis early allows patients and their caregivers to educate themselves about the disease and explore various management strategies. This knowledge empowers individuals to actively participate in their care, making informed decisions about nutrition, exercise, and therapy options. Early intervention can also provide access to support resources, including community support groups and caregiver networks, which can be invaluable for emotional and practical assistance throughout the disease journey.

Nutrition and diet play a significant role in managing Parkinson's symptoms. Early identification of the disease can prompt patients to modify their diets to include foods that support brain health and overall well-being. A nutrient-rich diet can help mitigate some symptoms associated with Parkinson's, such as fatigue and cognitive decline. Engaging with healthcare professionals early on can lead to personalized dietary recommendations that consider both the patient's preferences and nutritional needs.

Exercise and physical therapy are essential components of managing Parkinson's disease. Early detection allows for the incorporation of physical activity into daily routines, which can enhance mobility, balance, and strength. Regular exercise has been shown to improve not only physical health but also mental health, reducing anxiety and depression often associated with the diagnosis. Physical therapists can work with patients to develop tailored exercise programs that address their specific symptoms and limitations, ultimately promoting independence and enhancing quality of life.

Finally, advances in Parkinson's disease research are continually evolving, providing hope for better treatment options and management strategies. Early detection enables patients to participate in clinical trials or research studies that could lead to groundbreaking therapies. By being proactive in recognizing symptoms and seeking early diagnosis, patients and caregivers can stay informed about the latest developments in research, embracing innovative approaches to care that contribute to a more promising future in managing Parkinson's disease.

Chapter 2: Recognizing Early Symptoms

Tremors and Shaking

Tremors and shaking are among the most recognizable symptoms of Parkinson's disease, often serving as early indicators of the condition. These involuntary movements can manifest in various ways, typically beginning in the hands, fingers, or even the jaw. Patients may notice a rhythmic tremor when they are at rest, which can diminish with purposeful movement. Understanding the nature of these tremors is crucial as they not only affect daily activities but also contribute to the emotional and psychological impact of the disease.

The mechanism behind tremors in Parkinson's disease is primarily related to the loss of dopamine-producing neurons in the brain. This deficiency leads to disruptions in the pathways that control movement and coordination. Patients often describe their experience of tremors as a constant reminder of their condition, which can trigger feelings of frustration or helplessness. It is essential for patients and caregivers to recognize these early signs, as they can facilitate timely consultations with healthcare professionals for appropriate assessment and management.

Diet and nutrition can play a supportive role in managing tremors and overall symptoms. Certain nutrients, such as antioxidants and omega-3 fatty acids, may help protect brain health and support neuronal function. Patients should focus on a balanced diet rich in fruits, vegetables, whole grains, and lean proteins while staying well-hydrated. Consulting with a nutritionist who specializes in Parkinson's disease can provide tailored dietary strategies that may alleviate some symptoms and improve quality of life.

Exercise and physical therapy are vital components in managing tremors and promoting mobility. Regular physical activity can enhance muscle strength, coordination, and balance, potentially reducing the severity of tremors. Specific exercises, such as tai chi and yoga, have been shown to improve motor function and increase body awareness. Engaging in a structured exercise program under the guidance of a physical therapist can empower patients to take an active role in their health and mitigate some of the challenges posed by tremors.

Support from the community and caregiver resources is invaluable for individuals experiencing tremors and other symptoms of Parkinson's disease. Joining support groups can provide a platform to share experiences and coping strategies, fostering a sense of belonging and understanding. Caregivers also play a crucial role in providing emotional support, helping patients manage their symptoms, and ensuring they remain engaged in activities that promote their well-being. By leveraging available resources, patients can navigate the complexities of Parkinson's with greater resilience and confidence.

Muscle Rigidity

Muscle rigidity is a hallmark symptom of Parkinson's disease that can significantly impact daily functioning and overall quality of life. This stiffness in muscles often manifests as an increase in resistance to passive movement, affecting both the limbs and the trunk. Patients may notice that their muscles feel unusually tight or tense, which can lead to limited range of motion and discomfort. This rigidity can make simple tasks, such as dressing, walking, or even turning in bed, more challenging. Recognizing this symptom early can help patients and caregivers implement strategies to manage it effectively.

The underlying mechanism of muscle rigidity in Parkinson's disease is related to changes in the brain's motor pathways. The loss of dopamine-producing neurons in the substantia nigra leads to an imbalance in the signals that regulate muscle movement. This disruption can cause the muscles to contract more than necessary, resulting in the rigidity experienced by patients. Understanding the neurological basis of this symptom is crucial for patients and caregivers as it underscores the importance of seeking medical advice and intervention promptly when symptoms begin to appear.

Addressing muscle rigidity often involves a combination of pharmacological and non-pharmacological approaches. Medications such as levodopa and other dopaminergic agents can help alleviate the stiffness by replenishing dopamine levels in the brain. In addition to medication, physical therapy plays a vital role in managing muscle rigidity. Tailored exercise programs that include stretching, strengthening, and range-of-motion exercises can significantly improve flexibility and reduce stiffness. Regular physical activity not only helps manage rigidity but also promotes overall health and well-being.

Nutrition also plays a critical role in managing muscle rigidity and overall symptoms of Parkinson's disease. A balanced diet rich in antioxidants, healthy fats, and anti-inflammatory foods can support brain health and may help mitigate some of the symptoms associated with Parkinson's. Incorporating foods high in omega-3 fatty acids, such as fish and flaxseeds, along with plenty of fruits and vegetables, can contribute to better muscle function and reduced inflammation. Staying hydrated is equally important, as proper hydration can help muscles perform optimally.

Support from caregivers and the community is essential for patients experiencing muscle rigidity. Caregivers can assist by helping patients with exercises and daily activities that may be affected by stiffness. Additionally, support groups provide a platform for sharing experiences and strategies to cope with this challenging symptom. Together with advances in research and alternative therapies, such as massage and acupuncture, patients can find effective ways to manage muscle rigidity, enhancing their quality of life as they navigate the complexities of Parkinson's disease.

Bradykinesia (Slowness of Movement)

Bradykinesia, or slowness of movement, is one of the hallmark symptoms of Parkinson's disease and can significantly impact daily life. This symptom may manifest as a gradual reduction in the speed and amplitude of voluntary movements. Patients might notice that tasks they once performed quickly, such as buttoning a shirt or walking, now take more time and effort. Bradykinesia is not merely about reduced speed; it also affects the fluidity and coordination of movements, making activities feel laborious and frustrating. Recognizing these changes early can aid in managing the progression of the disease.

The mechanisms behind bradykinesia are rooted in the neurological changes associated with Parkinson's disease. The degeneration of dopamine-producing neurons in the brain leads to a disruption in the brain's ability to control movement. This lack of dopamine results in a slowed response to stimuli, making it challenging for patients to initiate or complete movements. Understanding this connection can help patients and caregivers recognize the importance of addressing bradykinesia early on, as it can serve as a critical indicator of disease progression.

Managing bradykinesia involves a multifaceted approach that includes exercise, nutrition, and possibly medication. Regular physical activity is essential, as it can enhance mobility, strength, and coordination. Engaging in activities like tai chi, yoga, and dance can help improve overall movement and flexibility. Nutrition also plays a vital role; a balanced diet rich in antioxidants and omega-3 fatty acids may support brain health and overall wellness. Patients should consult with healthcare professionals to develop a tailored regimen that addresses their specific needs.

Physical therapy can be particularly beneficial for those experiencing bradykinesia. A physical therapist can work with patients to implement exercises specifically designed to improve movement speed and coordination. Techniques such as "big movements" training, which encourages patients to exaggerate their movements, can be effective in overcoming the hesitance associated with bradykinesia. Additionally, occupational therapy can assist in adapting daily tasks to make them easier and less time-consuming, thus improving the quality of life for patients.

Support from caregivers and community resources is invaluable for managing bradykinesia and Parkinson's disease as a whole. Caregivers should be educated about the challenges associated with bradykinesia, enabling them to provide appropriate assistance and encouragement. Community support groups can offer a platform for patients and caregivers to share experiences, coping strategies, and resources. Together, these elements create a comprehensive support system that empowers patients to navigate the complexities of Parkinson's disease while addressing the challenges posed by bradykinesia.

Changes in Posture and Balance

Changes in posture and balance are among the early signs of Parkinson's Disease that patients and caregivers should recognize. As the disease progresses, individuals may experience a shift in their center of gravity, which can lead to a stooped posture and difficulty maintaining an upright position. This change is often subtle at first, but it can significantly impact daily activities and overall quality of life. Understanding these changes can help patients adapt their routines and seek appropriate interventions to manage their symptoms effectively.

One of the most common manifestations of posture changes in Parkinson's patients is the tendency to lean forward while walking. This forward tilt can create an imbalance that increases the risk of falls, a major concern for individuals with Parkinson's. Patients may find themselves shuffling their feet or taking smaller steps, which can further exacerbate balance issues. It is crucial for patients to be aware of these alterations and to communicate them to their healthcare providers, who can recommend strategies to improve posture and stability.

Physical therapy plays a vital role in addressing changes in posture and balance. Specialized exercises can strengthen core muscles, enhance flexibility, and improve coordination. Therapists may incorporate balance training into their sessions, helping patients develop techniques to stabilize themselves during movement. Engaging in regular physical activity not only addresses physical changes but also contributes to mental well-being. Caregivers should encourage patients to participate in these therapeutic exercises, fostering a supportive environment that promotes independence and confidence.

Nutrition also plays a critical role in managing the physical aspects of Parkinson's Disease. A well-balanced diet rich in vitamins and minerals can support muscle strength and overall health. Certain nutrients, such as omega-3 fatty acids and antioxidants, may help reduce inflammation and promote brain health, potentially mitigating some of the symptoms associated with changes in posture and balance. Caregivers can assist patients in making dietary choices that align with their health needs, ensuring they receive adequate nourishment to support their physical activities.

Finally, community support groups offer valuable resources for individuals experiencing changes in posture and balance due to Parkinson's Disease. These groups provide a platform for sharing experiences, strategies, and coping mechanisms among peers facing similar challenges. Engaging with others who understand the nuances of living with Parkinson's can empower patients and caregivers alike, fostering a sense of belonging and shared purpose. By raising awareness about these early signs and promoting proactive management, we can enhance the quality of life for those affected by Parkinson's Disease.

Non-Motor Symptoms

Non-motor symptoms of Parkinson's disease can often be overlooked, yet they significantly impact the quality of life for patients. While the hallmark motor symptoms such as tremors, stiffness, and bradykinesia are well recognized, non-motor symptoms can manifest in various ways, affecting emotional well-being, cognitive function, and even sleep patterns. Understanding these symptoms is crucial for patients and caregivers alike, as early recognition can lead to more effective management strategies and improved overall care.

One common non-motor symptom is depression, which affects a substantial number of individuals with Parkinson's disease. This can occur independently of the disease's progression and can significantly diminish motivation and energy levels. Patients might experience feelings of sadness, hopelessness, or a loss of interest in activities they once enjoyed. It is vital for patients to communicate openly with their healthcare providers about any mood changes, as effective treatment options, including therapy and medication, can greatly enhance emotional well-being.

Cognitive changes are another critical area of concern. Many patients report difficulties with memory, attention, and executive functions, which can lead to challenges in daily activities. These cognitive symptoms may not be immediately associated with Parkinson's, leading to frustration and confusion. Caregivers should be aware of these changes and encourage patients to engage in cognitive exercises and activities that promote mental stimulation. Additionally, discussing any cognitive concerns with healthcare providers can help in developing a tailored approach to manage these symptoms.

Sleep disturbances are prevalent among Parkinson's patients, with insomnia, restless legs syndrome, and excessive daytime sleepiness being common complaints. These issues can exacerbate other symptoms and contribute to fatigue, making it essential to address sleep hygiene and establish a consistent sleep routine. Simple lifestyle modifications, such as reducing screen time before bed, maintaining a comfortable sleep environment, and avoiding caffeine in the evening, can make a significant difference. In some cases, medical intervention may be necessary to address more severe sleep issues.

Finally, autonomic dysfunction, which includes symptoms such as constipation, urinary urgency, and orthostatic hypotension, can severely impact daily life. These symptoms are often underreported due to embarrassment or lack of awareness, but they can significantly affect both physical comfort and mental health. Patients should be encouraged to discuss these issues with their healthcare team to explore management options, including dietary adjustments, hydration strategies, and medications that may provide relief. By recognizing and addressing non-motor symptoms, patients and caregivers can work together to enhance the overall quality of life and navigate the challenges of Parkinson's disease more effectively.

Chapter 3: Nutrition and Diet for Parkinson's Patients

Importance of a Balanced Diet

A balanced diet plays a crucial role in the overall health and well-being of individuals with Parkinson's disease. Research suggests that a well-rounded nutritional approach can help manage symptoms, improve quality of life, and potentially slow disease progression. This is particularly important for patients who may experience challenges with digestion, appetite, and energy levels. By prioritizing a variety of foods that provide essential nutrients, Parkinson's patients can address specific dietary needs that arise from the condition and its treatment.

Key components of a balanced diet include a mix of fruits, vegetables, whole grains, lean proteins, and healthy fats. These food groups supply vital vitamins, minerals, and antioxidants that can support brain health and reduce inflammation. For instance, leafy greens and berries are known for their neuroprotective properties, which can be beneficial for cognitive function. Additionally, incorporating omega-3 fatty acids found in fish and flaxseeds may help with mood regulation, which is particularly important given the mental health challenges that can accompany Parkinson's disease.

Hydration is another critical element of a balanced diet that should not be overlooked. Many Parkinson's patients experience symptoms such as dry mouth and difficulties swallowing, which can make it harder to consume adequate fluids. Staying hydrated helps maintain energy levels, supports cognitive function, and aids in digestion. Caregivers and patients alike should focus on strategies to increase fluid intake, such as offering water-rich foods like fruits and soups, and ensuring that beverages are easily accessible and appealing.

Understanding the relationship between diet and medication is also vital for Parkinson's patients. Certain foods can interact with medications, affecting their efficacy. For instance, protein-rich foods may interfere with the absorption of levodopa, a common medication for Parkinson's symptoms. Therefore, patients should work closely with healthcare providers and nutritionists to create meal plans that optimize medication effectiveness while still providing balanced nutrition. This individualized approach can significantly enhance symptom management and overall health.

Finally, a balanced diet can foster a sense of community and support among patients and their caregivers. Sharing meals and recipes can strengthen social connections, which are essential for mental health. Community support groups often emphasize the importance of nutrition, and patients are encouraged to participate in discussions about dietary habits and experiences. By fostering an environment where dietary choices are shared and celebrated, patients can feel empowered in their journey, ultimately contributing to a holistic approach to managing Parkinson's disease.

Foods to Include

In managing Parkinson's disease, diet plays a crucial role in overall health and well-being. Foods rich in antioxidants, such as fruits and vegetables, can combat oxidative stress that may contribute to neurodegeneration. Berries, leafy greens, and cruciferous vegetables are particularly beneficial, as they contain high levels of vitamins C and E, which have been linked to improved brain health. Incorporating a variety of colors in your meals ensures a broad spectrum of nutrients, which is essential for maintaining energy levels and supporting neurological function.

In addition to antioxidants, omega-3 fatty acids are vital for individuals with Parkinson's. These healthy fats, found in fish like salmon, walnuts, and flaxseeds, have anti-inflammatory properties and may help protect brain cells from damage. Research suggests that omega-3s can enhance cognitive function and potentially slow the progression of Parkinson's symptoms. For those who prefer plant-based sources, incorporating chia seeds and hemp seeds into smoothies or salads can be an effective way to increase omega-3 intake.

Fiber-rich foods are also important for managing Parkinson's disease, particularly to alleviate constipation, a common symptom among patients. Whole grains, legumes, fruits, and vegetables not only provide fiber but also support digestive health. Foods such as oats, beans, and bran cereals can help maintain regular bowel movements while contributing essential nutrients to your diet. Staying hydrated is equally crucial, so pairing high-fiber foods with plenty of water can further enhance digestive function.

Moreover, incorporating fermented foods into your diet can positively influence gut health, which is increasingly recognized for its connection to brain health. Probiotic-rich foods like yogurt, kefir, sauerkraut, and kimchi may improve gut microbiota balance, potentially alleviating some Parkinson's symptoms. These foods can aid in digestion and enhance nutrient absorption, ensuring that your body receives the maximum benefits from the foods you eat.

Lastly, it is important to consider the role of hydration in managing Parkinson's disease. Proper fluid intake is vital for overall health, as dehydration can exacerbate symptoms such as fatigue and cognitive decline. Aim to drink water consistently throughout the day, and consider incorporating fluids from fruits and soups into your diet. By focusing on a balanced and varied diet that includes these essential foods, individuals with Parkinson's can support their health and improve their quality of life.

Foods to Avoid

Foods to avoid when managing Parkinson's disease play a crucial role in maintaining health and well-being. Certain dietary choices can exacerbate symptoms or interfere with medication efficacy. For individuals with Parkinson's, it is essential to be aware of specific foods that may impact their condition. High-protein foods, for instance, can interfere with the absorption of certain Parkinson's medications, particularly levodopa. While protein is an important part of a balanced diet, patients may consider timing their protein intake to ensure maximum medication effectiveness, often consuming proteins in the evening rather than with meals that include their medication.

Processed foods also warrant caution. These often contain high levels of sodium, unhealthy fats, and preservatives that can contribute to inflammation and overall poor health. Inflammatory responses can aggravate the symptoms of Parkinson's, making it vital for patients to focus on whole, unprocessed foods. Furthermore, processed snacks and fast foods can lead to weight gain, which may complicate mobility and overall fitness, important factors in managing Parkinson's disease effectively.

Additionally, foods high in sugar can lead to fluctuations in energy levels and mood, which can be problematic for those dealing with Parkinson's. Excessive sugar intake may promote inflammation and has been linked to various health complications, including cognitive decline. Opting for natural sources of sweetness, like fruits, can provide necessary nutrients without the adverse effects associated with refined sugars. This approach not only supports overall health but also helps maintain stable energy levels throughout the day.

Caffeine and alcohol consumption should also be approached with caution. While moderate caffeine may offer some benefits, excessive intake can lead to increased anxiety and sleep disturbances, both of which can worsen Parkinson's symptoms. Alcohol, on the other hand, can interact with medications and exacerbate balance issues, increasing the risk of falls. Patients should consult with healthcare providers to determine safe levels of these substances based on their individual health profiles.

Finally, foods that are difficult to chew or swallow can pose significant challenges for individuals with Parkinson's disease, especially as symptoms progress. Hard, crunchy, or sticky foods may lead to choking hazards or discomfort during meals. It is advisable to focus on softer, easier-to-manage foods that are still nutritious, such as smoothies, purees, and well-cooked vegetables. A mindful approach to diet can help improve quality of life for Parkinson's patients, making it essential to recognize and avoid foods that may hinder their health and symptom management.

Hydration and Its Role

Hydration is a crucial aspect of overall health, especially for individuals living with Parkinson's disease. Adequate fluid intake supports numerous bodily functions, including digestion, circulation, and temperature regulation. For Parkinson's patients, maintaining proper hydration can significantly impact their daily functioning and quality of life. Dehydration can exacerbate symptoms such as fatigue, confusion, and motor difficulties, making it essential to establish a routine that prioritizes fluid consumption.

The recommended daily water intake can vary based on factors such as age, weight, activity level, and individual health needs. For Parkinson's patients, it is vital to monitor their hydration closely, as some may experience changes in thirst sensation or difficulties in swallowing, known as dysphagia. Caregivers and loved ones can play an essential role in encouraging regular fluid intake by providing a variety of hydrating options, which can include water, herbal teas, and hydrating foods like fruits and vegetables.

In addition to traditional hydration methods, the role of nutrition in supporting hydration cannot be overlooked. Foods with high water content, such as cucumbers, tomatoes, and watermelon, can contribute to overall fluid intake. Moreover, incorporating electrolyte-rich beverages can help maintain the balance of fluids and minerals in the body. It is beneficial for Parkinson's patients to work with a nutritionist familiar with their unique needs to create a balanced diet that emphasizes both hydration and nutritional adequacy.

Exercise and physical therapy are also integral components of managing Parkinson's disease, and they can be positively influenced by hydration. Staying well-hydrated can improve energy levels, enhance physical performance, and alleviate some symptoms like muscle cramps and rigidity. Engaging in regular physical activity can stimulate thirst and encourage fluid consumption, making it a vital part of a holistic approach to care for those with Parkinson's.

Finally, the mental health implications of hydration should not be underestimated. Dehydration can lead to mood swings, irritability, and cognitive decline, which can be particularly concerning for Parkinson's patients who may already face challenges related to mental health. Community support groups can offer shared strategies for maintaining hydration, and caregivers can help create an environment that fosters regular fluid intake. By collectively prioritizing hydration, patients and caregivers can work together to enhance overall well-being and improve the management of Parkinson's disease.

Supplements and Nutritional Support

Supplements and nutritional support can play a significant role in managing Parkinson's disease, particularly in the early stages when patients may begin to notice subtle changes in their health. A well-rounded diet rich in essential nutrients can help bolster overall well-being and support brain health. Key nutrients such as omega-3 fatty acids, antioxidants, and certain vitamins and minerals are often highlighted in discussions about dietary strategies for neuroprotection. Incorporating foods such as fatty fish, leafy greens, nuts, and berries into daily meals may provide the necessary building blocks to help mitigate some of the symptoms associated with Parkinson's.

In addition to a balanced diet, some patients may consider dietary supplements to further enhance their nutritional intake. Supplements such as vitamin D, Coenzyme Q10, and B vitamins have garnered attention for their potential benefits in supporting neurological function and overall health. However, it is crucial to consult with healthcare providers before starting any new supplements, as interactions with medications or individual health conditions may occur. Personalized advice from a nutritionist or dietitian familiar with Parkinson's disease can also provide valuable insights into the most beneficial options.

Hydration is another vital component of nutritional support for Parkinson's patients. Many individuals may experience changes in swallowing or gastrointestinal function, which can affect fluid intake. Staying adequately hydrated is essential for maintaining energy levels, preventing constipation, and supporting cognitive function. Patients should aim to consume enough fluids throughout the day, and caregivers can assist by encouraging regular water intake and incorporating hydrating foods like fruits and soups into the diet.

Moreover, the role of nutrition extends beyond physical health; it also significantly impacts mental well-being. Research suggests that there is a connection between diet and mood, with certain foods potentially influencing mental health outcomes. For instance, diets high in processed foods and sugars may exacerbate feelings of depression or anxiety, which are common among those navigating the challenges of Parkinson's disease. Emphasizing whole foods and a balanced intake can contribute to a more stable mood and improved quality of life.

Finally, community support groups can provide a platform for sharing experiences and strategies related to nutrition and supplements. Engaging with others who are facing similar challenges can foster a sense of belonging and provide practical tips for meal planning, cooking, and navigating dietary changes. These groups often have resources available, including workshops or guest speakers on nutrition, which can further empower patients and caregivers in making informed dietary choices that support overall health and well-being in the context of Parkinson's disease.

Chapter 4: Exercise and Physical Therapy for Parkinson's

Benefits of Physical Activity

Physical activity offers numerous benefits for individuals living with Parkinson's disease, particularly in the early stages when symptoms may first present. Engaging in regular exercise can enhance motor function, improve balance, and reduce the risk of falls, which are critical factors for maintaining independence. Studies have shown that consistent physical activity helps to counteract the rigidity and bradykinesia commonly associated with Parkinson's, allowing patients to navigate daily tasks with greater ease and confidence.

Moreover, physical activity has a profound impact on mental health, which is especially important for those facing the challenges of a Parkinson's diagnosis. Exercise has been linked to reductions in anxiety and depression, providing a natural boost to mood and overall emotional well-being. The release of endorphins during physical activity can help mitigate feelings of sadness or frustration, enabling patients to maintain a more positive outlook on their health and future. This emotional resilience is vital in coping with the evolving nature of Parkinson's disease.

In addition to improving physical and mental health, physical activity plays a crucial role in enhancing cognitive function. Research indicates that regular exercise may help preserve cognitive abilities and even promote neuroprotection in individuals with Parkinson's. Engaging in activities that require coordination and concentration, such as dancing or tai chi, stimulates brain activity and can lead to improved memory and executive function. This cognitive engagement is essential for maintaining quality of life and supporting daily decision-making processes.

Social interaction is another significant benefit of participating in physical activities. Group exercise classes or community sports can foster connections with others who share similar experiences, helping to combat feelings of isolation that may accompany a Parkinson's diagnosis. These social bonds not only provide emotional support but also encourage individuals to stay active and committed to their exercise routines. Joining a community support group focused on physical activity can be an excellent way to build a network of friends and allies who understand the journey of living with Parkinson's.

Lastly, integrating physical activity into daily life can empower patients by giving them a sense of control over their health. Establishing and adhering to a personalized exercise regimen can lead to improved confidence and self-efficacy. As patients notice positive changes in their physical capabilities and overall well-being, they may feel more motivated to take an active role in managing their condition. This sense of empowerment is vital for navigating the complexities of Parkinson's disease and can significantly enhance the overall quality of life for individuals and their caregivers alike.

Recommended Types of Exercise

Engaging in regular physical activity is crucial for individuals living with Parkinson's disease, as it can help manage symptoms, improve mobility, and enhance overall quality of life. Several types of exercise have been shown to be particularly beneficial for those with early signs of the disease. These include aerobic exercises, strength training, flexibility exercises, balance training, and recreational activities. Each type serves distinct purposes and can be tailored to meet the varying needs and abilities of patients.

Aerobic exercises, such as walking, swimming, and cycling, can significantly improve cardiovascular health and overall endurance. These activities increase heart rate and promote better blood circulation, which is essential for maintaining energy levels and reducing fatigue. For those with Parkinson's, engaging in aerobic exercise for at least 150 minutes a week can lead to improvements in both physical and mental well-being. It's important to start at a comfortable pace and gradually increase intensity, ensuring that the exercise remains enjoyable and manageable.

Strength training is another vital component of an effective exercise regimen for Parkinson's patients. This type of exercise focuses on building muscle strength and can be performed using free weights, resistance bands, or body-weight exercises. Stronger muscles contribute to better posture, stability, and mobility, helping to counteract common symptoms such as rigidity and weakness. Even simple exercises targeting major muscle groups can yield significant benefits. It is advisable to work with a physical therapist or a qualified trainer to develop a safe and effective strength training program.

Flexibility exercises, including stretching and yoga, play a key role in maintaining joint health and preventing stiffness. These exercises enhance the range of motion and help alleviate some of the rigidity associated with Parkinson's disease. Incorporating flexibility routines into daily practice can improve balance and coordination, which are critical for reducing the risk of falls. Additionally, mindfulness practices such as yoga can also contribute to mental health by promoting relaxation and reducing anxiety, common challenges faced by individuals living with this condition.

Balance training is particularly important for Parkinson's patients, as they are at a higher risk of falls. Exercises that improve balance, such as tai chi and specific stability exercises, can enhance proprioception and coordination. Engaging in these activities not only boosts confidence in movement but also fosters independence in daily living. Recreational activities such as dancing, gardening, or even group sports can also provide social interaction and motivation, making exercise a more enjoyable and fulfilling part of life. For optimal results, it is recommended to combine various types of exercises and to consult with healthcare professionals to create a personalized exercise plan that takes into account individual capabilities and preferences.

Creating an Exercise Routine

Creating an exercise routine is a vital step for individuals experiencing early signs of Parkinson's disease. Regular physical activity can help manage symptoms, improve mobility, and enhance overall quality of life. When designing an exercise routine, it is essential to consider individual capabilities and preferences, ensuring that the chosen activities are safe, enjoyable, and tailored to personal needs. Consulting with healthcare professionals, such as physical therapists or exercise physiologists familiar with Parkinson's, can provide valuable insights into what types of exercises are most beneficial.

Incorporating a variety of exercise types can address different aspects of physical health. Aerobic exercises, such as walking, cycling, or swimming, can enhance cardiovascular fitness and endurance. Strength training is also crucial, as it helps to build muscle strength, which is often compromised in Parkinson's patients. Flexibility and balance exercises, such as yoga or tai chi, can improve posture, reduce stiffness, and decrease the risk of falls, a common concern for those with Parkinson's disease. A well-rounded routine should combine these elements for comprehensive benefits.

Establishing a consistent schedule is key to maintaining an effective exercise routine. Aim for at least 150 minutes of moderate-intensity aerobic activity each week, broken down into manageable sessions. This could mean engaging in 30 minutes of exercise five times a week, with additional strength training exercises included two to three times a week. Keeping track of progress can provide motivation and a sense of accomplishment. Consider using a journal or mobile app to monitor activities and any improvements in physical capabilities or symptoms.

Social support can play a significant role in adherence to an exercise routine. Joining community support groups or exercise classes specifically designed for individuals with Parkinson's can foster a sense of camaraderie and encourage regular participation. Exercising with others not only enhances motivation but also provides an opportunity to share experiences and strategies for coping with the disease. Caregivers can also benefit from being involved in these activities, as they can better understand the needs of their loved ones while enhancing their own well-being.

Adapting exercises as the disease progresses is crucial for safety and effectiveness. Regularly reassessing the routine and making modifications based on changing abilities will ensure that the exercises remain beneficial and engaging. It is also important to listen to the body and rest when needed, as fatigue can impact performance and overall health. By prioritizing an adaptable and enjoyable exercise routine, individuals with early signs of Parkinson's disease can take proactive steps toward better managing their health and maintaining a higher quality of life.

Working with a Physical Therapist

Working with a physical therapist can be a transformative experience for individuals navigating the early signs of Parkinson's Disease. Physical therapy focuses on improving mobility, strength, and overall physical function, which can be particularly beneficial as the disease progresses. Early intervention through tailored exercise regimens can help mitigate some of the motor symptoms associated with Parkinson's, such as rigidity, bradykinesia, and postural instability. It is essential to find a physical therapist who has experience working with Parkinson's patients, as they will be familiar with the unique challenges posed by the disease.

During the initial sessions, the physical therapist will typically conduct a comprehensive assessment. This evaluation may include a review of your medical history, an assessment of your current physical abilities, and a discussion of your specific goals and concerns. The therapist will consider factors such as balance, coordination, strength, and flexibility, which are critical in developing a personalized treatment plan. This plan may include exercises designed to enhance muscle strength, improve balance, and promote overall endurance, tailored specifically to your capabilities and comfort level.

As you progress with your physical therapy sessions, it is crucial to communicate openly with your therapist about your experiences and any changes in your condition. Parkinson's can present differently for each person, and your feedback will help the therapist adjust your program as needed. They may incorporate various techniques such as stretching, resistance training, and gait training. Additionally, they might introduce activities that focus on enhancing daily living skills, which can help maintain independence and improve your quality of life.

Incorporating physical therapy into your routine can also provide psychological benefits. Engaging in regular physical activity can boost mood, reduce anxiety, and alleviate feelings of isolation that many Parkinson's patients experience. Furthermore, working with a therapist can foster a sense of community and support, as they often encourage participation in group therapy sessions or wellness activities. This social interaction can be invaluable in building relationships with others facing similar challenges.

Finally, it is essential to recognize that physical therapy is most effective when combined with a holistic approach to managing Parkinson's. This may include nutritional support, alternative therapies, and caregiver involvement. By working closely with your physical therapist and incorporating their recommendations into your daily life, you can create a comprehensive management plan that addresses both the physical and emotional aspects of living with Parkinson's Disease. Emphasizing collaboration among healthcare providers, caregivers, and support groups can lead to improved outcomes and a more empowered approach to navigating the early signs of the disease.

Safety Considerations

Safety considerations are paramount for individuals navigating the early signs of Parkinson's disease. As symptoms may include tremors, rigidity, and balance issues, it is crucial to create a safe living environment. This involves assessing the home for potential hazards such as loose rugs, cluttered walkways, and inadequate lighting. Simple modifications, like securing rugs with non-slip pads or removing obstacles, can significantly reduce the risk of falls. Additionally, ensuring that commonly used items are within easy reach can help minimize the need for unnecessary movements that might lead to accidents.

In the context of nutrition and diet, safety also extends to food preparation and consumption. Patients may experience difficulties with fine motor skills, making meal preparation challenging. Utilizing adaptive kitchen tools can enhance safety and independence. Moreover, it is important to consider food consistency, as some individuals may have swallowing difficulties. Consulting with a healthcare provider or a registered dietitian can provide tailored advice on creating a safe and nutritious meal plan that accommodates these needs.

Exercise and physical therapy play a vital role in maintaining safety for Parkinson's patients. Regular physical activity can improve strength, balance, and coordination, thereby reducing the risk of falls. Engaging in supervised exercise programs specifically designed for individuals with Parkinson's can ensure that activities are safe and effective. Physical therapists can also teach patients how to fall safely, which can help mitigate injuries in the event of a fall. Furthermore, incorporating assistive devices, such as canes or walkers, can provide additional support during physical activities.

Caregiver support is another crucial aspect of safety considerations. Caregivers should be educated about the symptoms of Parkinson's and trained in proper techniques to assist with mobility and daily tasks. This training can help prevent caregiver injuries while ensuring that patients receive the necessary support. Open communication between caregivers and patients is essential to understand the patient's needs and preferences, fostering a safe environment that promotes independence while ensuring assistance is available when required.

Lastly, mental health is a significant aspect of overall safety for Parkinson's patients. Anxiety and depression can exacerbate physical symptoms and affect decision-making, which may lead to unsafe situations. It is vital to prioritize mental health through support groups, therapy, and community engagement. Establishing connections with others facing similar challenges can provide emotional support and practical advice on navigating daily life with Parkinson's. Integrating mental health care into the overall treatment plan can enhance safety and quality of life for individuals living with Parkinson's disease.

Chapter 5: Caregiver Support and Resources for Parkinson's

Understanding the Caregiver's Role

Understanding the caregiver's role is essential in the management and support of individuals living with Parkinson's disease. Caregivers often become the primary source of assistance, providing emotional support, physical help, and advocacy for their loved ones. This role can encompass a range of responsibilities, from assisting with daily activities such as dressing and bathing to managing medications and coordinating medical appointments. Recognizing the complexity of this role can empower caregivers to seek appropriate resources and support, ensuring both their well-being and that of the person they care for.

The emotional landscape of caregiving is significant, as caregivers frequently experience a mix of stress, compassion, and fulfillment. Understanding the nuances of these emotions is crucial. Caregivers may face feelings of frustration and helplessness, especially as they navigate the challenges of Parkinson's disease, which can include fluctuations in mobility and changes in cognitive function. Acknowledging these feelings and allowing for open communication can foster a more supportive environment for both the caregiver and the patient. It is important for caregivers to engage in self-care practices and seek out support networks to address their emotional needs.

Practical knowledge about Parkinson's disease and its progression can greatly enhance a caregiver's effectiveness. Familiarization with early symptoms, such as tremors, rigidity, and changes in posture, allows caregivers to recognize when additional support may be necessary. Moreover, understanding the disease's impact on daily living can inform the development of routines that promote independence and dignity for the patient. Caregivers are often in the best position to observe changes in behavior or physical condition, making their insights valuable to healthcare providers.

Nutrition and exercise are critical components in the management of Parkinson's disease, and caregivers play a significant role in facilitating these aspects. A well-balanced diet can help optimize the patient's health and manage symptoms, while regular physical activity can improve mobility and overall quality of life. Caregivers can assist in planning meals that align with dietary recommendations and encourage participation in suitable exercise programs. Knowledge of community resources, such as local support groups and physical therapy options, can further enhance the caregiver's ability to provide comprehensive support.

Finally, caregivers should be aware of the importance of advocacy and staying informed about advances in Parkinson's disease research and treatment options. This includes understanding alternative therapies and assistive technologies that may benefit the patient. By being proactive and informed, caregivers can advocate effectively for their loved ones, ensuring they receive the best possible care. Engaging with community support groups not only provides caregivers with valuable information but also offers a sense of camaraderie and shared experience, reinforcing the vital role they play in the lives of those living with Parkinson's disease.

Emotional and Physical Support for Caregivers

Emotional and physical support for caregivers is vital in the context of Parkinson's disease, where the demands on caregivers can be significant. Caregivers often face a range of challenges, including managing daily tasks, providing emotional reassurance, and adapting to the changing needs of the person with Parkinson's. Understanding these challenges is crucial for both caregivers and patients, as it fosters a supportive environment that can enhance the quality of life for everyone involved.

One important aspect of caregiver support is emotional well-being. Caregivers may experience feelings of stress, anxiety, and even depression as they navigate the complexities of providing care. It is essential to encourage caregivers to seek support through counseling or support groups tailored for those caring for individuals with Parkinson's. These resources can provide a safe space for caregivers to share experiences, gain insights, and develop coping strategies, ultimately helping them manage their emotional health more effectively.

Physical support is equally important, as caregivers often take on physically demanding tasks. This can include assisting with mobility, managing household chores, and providing personal care. Implementing adaptive techniques and utilizing assistive technologies can significantly reduce the physical strain on caregivers. Simple modifications at home, such as installing grab bars or using mobility aids, can enhance safety and ease the caregiving process, allowing caregivers to focus more on emotional connections and less on physical limitations.

Nutrition also plays a crucial role in sustaining caregivers' energy levels and overall health. A balanced diet can help caregivers maintain their physical strength and mental clarity, which is essential in managing the demands of caregiving. Encouraging caregivers to prioritize their nutrition, engage in regular exercise, and take breaks can help mitigate the risk of burnout. Caregivers should also be reminded that self-care is not selfish; it is a necessary component of providing effective care.

Lastly, fostering a community of support can greatly enhance the experience of caregiving. Connecting with other caregivers through local support groups or online forums can create a sense of camaraderie and shared understanding. These connections can provide valuable insights into effective caregiving practices and emotional support during challenging times. By recognizing the importance of emotional and physical support for caregivers, we can better navigate the complexities of Parkinson's disease together, ensuring both caregivers and patients experience a higher quality of life.

Resources and Organizations for Caregivers

Caregiving for individuals with Parkinson's disease can be both rewarding and challenging. Recognizing the complexities involved, it is essential for caregivers to have access to resources and organizations that can provide support and information. Many organizations focus specifically on Parkinson's disease, offering educational materials, guidance, and assistance to both patients and their caregivers. These resources help caregivers better understand the disease, its progression, and effective strategies for managing symptoms.

One notable organization is the Parkinson's Foundation, which provides a wealth of information, including care planning guides, medication management tools, and tips for effective communication with healthcare providers. They also offer local support groups and educational events that allow caregivers to connect with others facing similar challenges. Accessing these resources can alleviate feelings of isolation and help caregivers develop skills to better support their loved ones.

Another significant resource is the Michael J. Fox Foundation for Parkinson's Research, which not only funds innovative research but also disseminates knowledge about the latest advancements in the field. This organization provides caregivers with updates on emerging therapies and clinical trials that may benefit their loved ones. Staying informed about research developments can empower caregivers and patients alike, offering hope and new options for managing the disease.

Local community support groups also play a crucial role in providing emotional support and practical advice. Many communities host regular meetings where caregivers can share experiences, discuss challenges, and learn from one another. These groups often invite healthcare professionals to speak on various topics related to Parkinson's disease, including nutrition, exercise, and mental health. This collaborative environment fosters a sense of camaraderie and understanding that can be invaluable in the caregiving journey.

In addition to these organizations, there are numerous online resources available that offer forums, webinars, and articles dedicated to caregiver support. Websites like Caregiver Action Network and AgingCare provide tools and tips for managing caregiving responsibilities, as well as information on self-care strategies to ensure caregivers maintain their own well-being. By utilizing these resources, caregivers can enhance their knowledge, access critical support, and ultimately improve the quality of life for both themselves and the individuals they care for.

Communication Strategies

Effective communication is crucial for individuals navigating the early signs of Parkinson's disease, as it impacts both the patient and their caregivers. Establishing clear communication strategies can help patients articulate their experiences and needs, while also enabling caregivers to provide appropriate support. One of the first steps in improving communication is to create an open environment where patients feel safe to express their feelings and concerns. This includes encouraging them to share their observations about symptoms, emotional states, and any changes in their daily routines. Active listening by caregivers and healthcare providers fosters trust and understanding, which are essential for effective communication.

Utilizing visual aids and technology can enhance communication for those experiencing difficulties due to Parkinson's disease. Many patients may face challenges such as slurred speech or diminished vocal volume, making it harder to communicate verbally. Integrating assistive technologies, like speech-to-text applications or communication boards, can bridge the gap. Visual aids can also support discussions about symptoms or treatment options, helping patients articulate their needs more effectively. By adopting these tools, caregivers can better understand the patient's condition and preferences, ensuring that their concerns are addressed promptly.

It is equally important to be mindful of non-verbal communication cues, which can often convey more than words themselves. Facial expressions, gestures, and body language play a significant role in how messages are communicated and received. For caregivers, being attuned to these non-verbal signals can provide valuable insights into a patient's emotional and physical state. This awareness can lead to more compassionate interactions and can help caregivers respond appropriately to unspoken needs, thereby enhancing the overall quality of care provided.

Regular check-ins can serve as a vital communication strategy, allowing for ongoing dialogue between patients and caregivers. Scheduled conversations can provide a structured way for patients to discuss their symptoms, treatment progress, and any concerns they might have. This proactive approach not only helps in early identification of any worsening symptoms but also reinforces the patient's autonomy and involvement in their care. Caregivers should ask open-ended questions to encourage patients to express themselves fully, leading to a more comprehensive understanding of their experience with the disease.

Finally, fostering a support network through community engagement can greatly enhance communication strategies for both patients and caregivers. Joining support groups provides an opportunity to share experiences and learn from others facing similar challenges. These groups often serve as safe spaces where patients can discuss their feelings and symptoms without fear of judgment. Additionally, engaging with community resources, such as nutrition and exercise programs tailored for Parkinson's patients, can facilitate dialogue around best practices for managing the disease. By embracing a holistic approach to communication, patients and caregivers can work together more effectively, leading to improved outcomes and a better quality of life.

Balancing Caregiving with Personal Life

Balancing caregiving with personal life is a crucial aspect of managing the complexities that come with Parkinson's disease. Caregivers often face the challenge of providing support while also ensuring that their own needs are met. It is essential for caregivers to recognize the signs of caregiver fatigue and stress, which can impact their ability to provide effective care. Establishing a routine that includes self-care practices is vital. This may involve setting aside time for hobbies, exercise, or simply moments of rest. Prioritizing personal well-being not only benefits the caregiver but also enhances the quality of care provided to the individual with Parkinson's.

Effective communication is a cornerstone of balancing caregiving and personal life. Caregivers should engage openly with the individual they are caring for, discussing needs, limitations, and expectations. Regular conversations can help clarify responsibilities and allow caregivers to express their feelings and concerns. Utilizing support networks, including family members, friends, or professional services, can alleviate some of the pressures faced by caregivers. By sharing responsibilities, caregivers can carve out time for themselves while ensuring that their loved one receives the attention they require.

Incorporating a structured schedule can also aid in achieving balance. Caregivers might find it beneficial to create a daily or weekly plan that outlines caregiving tasks alongside personal commitments. This approach not only helps in managing time efficiently but also minimizes the feeling of being overwhelmed. It is advisable to remain flexible within that schedule, as unexpected challenges may arise in the caregiving process. Planning for these contingencies can reduce stress and provide caregivers with a sense of control over their situation.

Exploring available resources for caregiver support can be incredibly beneficial. Numerous organizations provide information, workshops, and support groups tailored specifically for caregivers of individuals with Parkinson's disease. Connecting with these resources can offer both practical assistance and emotional support. Engaging with community support groups can provide a sense of camaraderie and understanding, as caregivers share their experiences and strategies for coping with the unique challenges they face. These connections can help alleviate feelings of isolation and foster a supportive environment.

Lastly, caregivers should embrace the idea that seeking help is a strength, not a weakness. It is important to recognize that balancing caregiving with personal life is an ongoing process that may require adjustments over time. Caregivers should not hesitate to reach out for professional support, whether through counseling or respite care services, to allow themselves the necessary breaks to recharge. By taking proactive steps to maintain their own health and well-being, caregivers can sustain their ability to provide compassionate and effective care, ultimately benefiting both themselves and the individuals they support.

Chapter 6: Advances in Parkinson's Disease Research

Current Research Trends

Current research trends in Parkinson's disease (PD) are increasingly focused on early detection, innovative treatments, and comprehensive management strategies. The understanding of PD has evolved significantly, shifting from traditional views of the disease as solely a movement disorder to a multi-faceted condition that affects various aspects of health, including cognitive functions, emotional well-being, and quality of life. Researchers are now exploring how early symptoms, such as subtle changes in motor skills, sense of smell, and sleep patterns, can serve as critical indicators for the onset of Parkinson's. Recognizing these signs early is essential for timely intervention and improved patient outcomes.

Nutrition and diet have emerged as vital components in the management of Parkinson's disease. Current studies are investigating the impact of specific dietary patterns and nutrients on disease progression and symptom management. For instance, there is growing evidence that diets rich in antioxidants and omega-3 fatty acids may have neuroprotective effects. Research is also focusing on how certain foods can influence medication absorption and efficacy, highlighting the importance of personalized nutrition plans for PD patients. By understanding nutritional needs, patients can potentially enhance their overall health and mitigate some symptoms associated with the disease.

Exercise and physical therapy are critical areas of focus in current Parkinson's research. Emerging studies are illustrating the profound impact of regular physical activity on mobility, balance, and overall quality of life for PD patients. Not only does exercise help in managing motor symptoms, but it also plays a key role in reducing depression and anxiety, which are common among individuals with Parkinson's. Innovative exercise programs, including dance, tai chi, and strength training, are being evaluated for their effectiveness in enhancing motor function and promoting mental well-being. The integration of physical therapy into treatment plans is becoming increasingly recognized as essential for maintaining independence and improving daily functioning.

Mental health is another significant area of research, as psychological well-being is closely linked to the overall health of Parkinson's patients. Studies are delving into the prevalence of anxiety, depression, and cognitive decline among those with PD, emphasizing the need for comprehensive mental health support. Current trends highlight the importance of integrating mental health resources into the care model for Parkinson's patients, ensuring that both physical and emotional needs are addressed. This holistic approach aims to provide a more rounded support system for patients and their caregivers, enabling them to navigate the complexities of living with Parkinson's disease.

Finally, advances in technology are transforming the landscape of Parkinson's disease management. Research is increasingly focusing on assistive technologies that can enhance the quality of life for patients. Wearable devices, mobile applications, and telehealth services are being developed to monitor symptoms, track medication adherence, and facilitate communication with healthcare providers. These technologies not only empower patients to take an active role in their care but also provide caregivers with valuable resources and support. As research continues to evolve, the integration of technology into Parkinson's care is expected to create new opportunities for improving patient outcomes and fostering a supportive community for those affected by the disease.

Clinical Trials and Their Importance

Clinical trials are essential for advancing our understanding of Parkinson's disease and improving the treatment landscape for those affected by it. These carefully designed research studies test new therapies, medications, and interventions, offering hope for better management of early symptoms and overall disease progression. For patients navigating the complexities of Parkinson's, participating in clinical trials can provide access to cutting-edge treatments that are not yet available on the market, as well as contribute to the broader understanding of the disease.

The importance of clinical trials lies not only in their potential to offer new treatment options but also in their role in validating existing therapies. Through rigorous testing and evaluation, clinical trials help identify which interventions are most effective in alleviating symptoms, enhancing quality of life, and addressing specific challenges faced by Parkinson's patients. This evidence-based approach ensures that patients receive therapies that have proven benefits, ultimately leading to better health outcomes.

For caregivers and family members, understanding clinical trials can be crucial in supporting their loved ones. Knowledge of ongoing studies can open up discussions about potential participation, allowing caregivers to help patients weigh the benefits and risks. Additionally, being informed about the latest research and findings can empower caregivers to advocate for their loved ones and make informed decisions regarding treatment options.

Patients should be aware that clinical trials often focus on various aspects of Parkinson's disease, including nutrition, exercise, and mental health. Some studies may explore how dietary interventions can affect symptom management, while others may investigate the impact of physical therapy and exercise regimens. These trials are vital for uncovering holistic approaches to care, which can significantly improve daily functioning and emotional well-being for individuals living with Parkinson's.

Finally, participating in clinical trials fosters a sense of community among patients, caregivers, and researchers. By joining these studies, patients become part of a collective effort to combat Parkinson's disease, sharing their experiences and contributing to vital research. This connection not only enhances the patient experience but also promotes a shared commitment to advancing knowledge and improving care for all those affected by Parkinson's.

Emerging Treatments and Therapies

Emerging treatments and therapies for Parkinson's Disease are evolving rapidly, providing new hope for patients navigating the complexities of this condition. Traditional approaches have focused primarily on medication, such as levodopa and dopamine agonists, to manage symptoms. However, ongoing research is leading to innovative therapies that target the underlying mechanisms of the disease. These advancements aim not only to alleviate symptoms but also to slow disease progression, offering a more holistic approach to treatment.

One promising area of research involves gene therapy, which seeks to address the genetic factors that may contribute to the onset and progression of Parkinson's Disease. By delivering genes that encode proteins essential for neuronal function, scientists hope to restore the balance of neurotransmitters in the brain. Early clinical trials have shown encouraging results, suggesting that gene therapy could potentially modify the course of the disease rather than merely treating its symptoms. As these studies advance, they could pave the way for personalized medicine tailored to the genetic profile of individual patients.

Another significant development is the exploration of neuroprotective agents that aim to shield neurons from degeneration. Compounds such as Nilotinib and other repurposed drugs are currently being investigated for their ability to enhance cellular resilience. These treatments focus on reducing oxidative stress and inflammation, both of which are implicated in the progression of Parkinson's. As research continues, the hope is that these neuroprotective strategies will provide patients with a more effective means of managing their condition over the long term.

Additionally, non-pharmacological therapies are gaining traction as essential components of comprehensive care for Parkinson's patients. Mindfulness-based interventions, cognitive behavioral therapy, and art therapy are being studied for their potential to improve mental health and overall quality of life. These approaches can help patients manage anxiety, depression, and other mental health issues commonly associated with Parkinson's, promoting emotional well-being alongside physical health. Integrating these therapies into treatment plans can create a more supportive environment for both patients and caregivers.

Lastly, advancements in assistive technologies are transforming daily living for many individuals with Parkinson's Disease. Devices designed to enhance mobility, communication, and daily tasks are becoming increasingly sophisticated, allowing patients to maintain independence for longer. Wearable technology can monitor movement patterns and provide real-time feedback, while smart home devices can simplify daily routines. As these technologies continue to develop, they promise to offer practical solutions that not only improve functionality but also enhance the overall quality of life for those affected by Parkinson's.

The Future of Parkinson's Disease Research

The future of Parkinson's Disease research is poised to reshape our understanding and management of this complex condition. With advances in technology and a deeper understanding of neurobiology, researchers are exploring new avenues that could lead to earlier diagnosis and more effective treatments. Innovations in imaging techniques, for instance, allow scientists to observe brain changes associated with Parkinson's at much earlier stages. This shift towards early intervention is critical, as it could significantly improve the quality of life for patients by enabling them to adopt proactive lifestyle changes and therapeutic strategies sooner.

Genetic research is also at the forefront of future developments in Parkinson's studies. With the identification of several genetic markers linked to the disease, there is growing potential for personalized medicine approaches. Understanding an individual's genetic predisposition to Parkinson's could lead to tailored treatment plans that address specific needs and risks. This could involve not only pharmacological interventions but also targeted dietary and exercise recommendations that align with the genetic profile of the patient, enhancing the effectiveness of management strategies.

Advances in assistive technologies continue to offer promising solutions for improving daily living for Parkinson's patients. Wearable devices that monitor movement and provide real-time feedback are already making a difference in how individuals manage their symptoms. Future developments may include sophisticated applications that integrate with smart home systems, enabling a more seamless interaction with the environment. These technologies can empower patients and caregivers, providing crucial support and resources that enhance independence and safety.

Research into alternative therapies is gaining traction, as many patients seek holistic approaches to managing their symptoms. Investigations into the efficacy of practices such as acupuncture, yoga, and dietary supplements are expanding. Future studies aim to clarify which alternative therapies are most beneficial and how they can be effectively integrated into conventional treatment plans. This holistic perspective not only addresses physical symptoms but also considers mental health, emphasizing the importance of emotional well-being in the overall management of Parkinson's Disease.

Community support and collaboration are essential components of future Parkinson's research. Initiatives that encourage patient and caregiver involvement in research processes are increasing, fostering a more inclusive environment. This collaborative approach can lead to the identification of real-world challenges faced by patients and caregivers, guiding research efforts towards solutions that have a meaningful impact. By engaging the community, researchers can ensure that the focus remains not only on scientific breakthroughs but also on improving the lived experiences of those affected by Parkinson's Disease.

Chapter 7: Alternative Therapies for Parkinson's Management

Overview of Alternative Therapies

Alternative therapies have gained traction as a complementary approach for managing Parkinson's disease, offering patients various methods to alleviate symptoms and enhance their quality of life. These therapies often focus on holistic well-being, addressing not just the physical aspects of the disease but also emotional and psychological needs. While they should not replace conventional medical treatments, alternative therapies can serve as valuable adjuncts, providing relief and empowerment for those navigating the complexities of Parkinson's.

Among the most recognized alternative therapies is acupuncture, which involves the insertion of thin needles into specific points on the body. Many patients report improvement in symptoms such as tremors, stiffness, and sleep disturbances after undergoing acupuncture sessions. This therapy is believed to help restore balance and promote relaxation, potentially enhancing the overall sense of well-being. Additionally, mindfulness practices, including meditation and yoga, have shown promise in reducing anxiety and stress, which can exacerbate Parkinson's symptoms.

Nutrition also plays a crucial role in managing Parkinson's disease, and dietary modifications may serve as an alternative therapy. Patients are encouraged to adopt a balanced diet rich in antioxidants, omega-3 fatty acids, and fiber to support brain health and manage symptoms. Some studies suggest that certain dietary patterns, such as the Mediterranean diet, may be beneficial for neuroprotection. Patients should work with nutritionists familiar with Parkinson's to develop personalized meal plans that cater to their needs and preferences.

Exercise and physical therapy are essential components of alternative therapies for Parkinson's management. Regular physical activity can help maintain mobility, balance, and strength, thereby reducing the risk of falls and improving overall function. Exercise programs tailored for Parkinson's patients often include activities like tai chi, dance, and resistance training, which not only enhance physical capabilities but also foster social connections. Engaging in group exercises can provide motivation and support, reinforcing the importance of community in managing the disease.

Lastly, the role of caregiver support and community resources cannot be overlooked in the context of alternative therapies. Caregivers often play a vital role in facilitating access to these therapies and providing emotional support. Support groups can offer a platform for sharing experiences and strategies, fostering a sense of belonging among patients and caregivers alike. By exploring alternative therapies, patients with Parkinson's disease can take an active role in their health management, benefiting from a comprehensive approach that addresses both physical and emotional dimensions.

Mind-Body Approaches

Mind-body approaches encompass a range of techniques that emphasize the connection between mental and physical health, particularly beneficial for individuals navigating the early signs of Parkinson's disease. These methods can help manage symptoms, improve overall well-being, and enhance the quality of life for patients. This subchapter explores various mind-body interventions, including mindfulness, meditation, yoga, and tai chi, which have shown promise in alleviating some of the challenges associated with Parkinson's.

Mindfulness practices involve paying attention to the present moment without judgment, which can reduce stress and anxiety levels. For Parkinson's patients, incorporating mindfulness into daily routines can foster a greater sense of control over their physical and emotional experiences. Studies indicate that mindfulness can lead to improvements in mood, cognitive function, and even motor symptoms, making it a valuable tool for managing the psychological aspects of the disease. Simple mindfulness exercises, such as deep breathing or guided imagery, can easily be integrated into the day-to-day activities of patients.

Meditation is another powerful mind-body technique that can offer significant benefits to individuals with Parkinson's disease. Engaging in regular meditation can reduce symptoms of anxiety and depression, both of which are common among Parkinson's patients. Different forms of meditation, such as loving-kindness or body scan meditation, can enhance emotional resilience and foster a greater sense of peace. Patients may find it helpful to join meditation groups, either in-person or online, where they can connect with others facing similar challenges and share techniques that work for them.

Yoga and tai chi are physical practices that also incorporate mindfulness and meditation elements, promoting physical flexibility, balance, and strength. These low-impact exercises can be particularly beneficial for Parkinson's patients, as they help improve mobility and reduce the risk of falls. Additionally, the community aspect of yoga and tai chi classes can provide essential social support for patients and caregivers alike. Many community centers and health facilities offer specialized classes designed for those living with Parkinson's, ensuring that participants receive appropriate guidance tailored to their needs.

Incorporating mind-body approaches into a holistic care plan can empower Parkinson's patients and their caregivers to take an active role in managing the disease. These techniques can complement traditional medical interventions and provide a sense of agency in the face of uncertainty. As research continues to evolve, exploring the effectiveness of mind-body approaches in the context of Parkinson's disease will be crucial. Patients are encouraged to discuss these options with their healthcare providers to create a comprehensive and personalized management plan that addresses both their physical and emotional health.

Acupuncture and Massage Therapy

Acupuncture and massage therapy are increasingly recognized as valuable complementary approaches for managing the symptoms of Parkinson's disease. These alternative therapies can help alleviate discomfort, improve mobility, and enhance overall well-being. For patients navigating early signs of Parkinson's, incorporating these techniques into a holistic care plan may provide additional relief from common symptoms such as stiffness, pain, and stress. Understanding the mechanisms behind acupuncture and massage can empower patients and caregivers to make informed decisions about their health management.

Acupuncture involves the insertion of fine needles into specific points on the body to stimulate energy flow, known as "Qi." Research suggests that acupuncture may help reduce muscle stiffness and improve motor function in Parkinson's patients. By promoting circulation and decreasing inflammation, acupuncture can also address non-motor symptoms such as anxiety and sleep disturbances. Patients who seek acupuncture should look for licensed practitioners experienced in treating neurological conditions to ensure safety and effectiveness.

Massage therapy, on the other hand, focuses on manipulating the soft tissues of the body to relieve tension and pain. Different types of massage, such as Swedish, deep tissue, and myofascial release, can be tailored to meet the unique needs of Parkinson's patients. Regular massage sessions may enhance flexibility and reduce muscle tightness, contributing to a better range of motion. Additionally, the emotional benefits of massage—such as relaxation and stress reduction—can be particularly beneficial for individuals dealing with the psychological impact of a Parkinson's diagnosis.

Combining acupuncture and massage therapy with conventional treatments can create a more comprehensive approach to managing Parkinson's symptoms. It is essential for patients to communicate openly with their healthcare providers about their interest in these therapies. This collaboration can help ensure that all aspects of care align and support the patient's overall treatment goals. Caregivers can also play a crucial role in facilitating access to these therapies, helping patients navigate appointments, and providing emotional support throughout the process.

As awareness of alternative therapies for Parkinson's continues to grow, community support groups can serve as valuable resources for patients seeking information and shared experiences. These groups often provide insights into local practitioners, personal success stories, and tips for integrating acupuncture and massage into daily routines. By connecting with others who understand their challenges, patients can gain motivation and encouragement to explore all available options for managing their symptoms and improving their quality of life.

Herbal Remedies and Supplements

Herbal remedies and supplements have gained popularity among individuals seeking complementary approaches to managing Parkinson's disease. While these natural options are not substitutes for conventional medical treatment, they may offer additional support in addressing some of the symptoms associated with Parkinson's. Many patients turn to herbs and supplements in hopes of improving their overall well-being, managing motor and non-motor symptoms, and enhancing their quality of life. It is essential, however, for patients to approach these remedies with caution and to consult healthcare professionals before integrating them into their treatment plans.

Several herbs have shown promise in research related to Parkinson's disease. For instance, Ginkgo biloba is often discussed for its potential to improve cognitive function and memory, which can be affected in Parkinson's patients. Similarly, turmeric, containing the active compound curcumin, is noted for its anti-inflammatory and antioxidant properties. These qualities may help mitigate some of the neurodegenerative processes seen in Parkinson's disease. Patients should consider the scientific evidence supporting these herbs and discuss their use with a healthcare provider to ensure they do not interfere with prescribed medications.

In addition to herbs, various dietary supplements are being explored for their potential benefits. Coenzyme Q10 is one such supplement that has garnered attention for its role in mitochondrial function and energy production, both of which can be compromised in Parkinson's disease. Omega-3 fatty acids, found in fish oil, are also recognized for their anti-inflammatory effects and their possible role in brain health. Other supplements, such as vitamin D and B vitamins, may support overall neurological health. Patients should be mindful of dosages and possible interactions with their current medications when considering these supplements.

It is also important for patients to recognize that not all herbal remedies and supplements are created equal. Quality and purity can vary significantly among products on the market. Patients should seek out reputable brands that provide third-party testing or certifications to ensure they are consuming safe and effective products. Engaging with a knowledgeable healthcare provider, such as a registered dietitian or a physician familiar with integrative medicine, can help patients make informed choices about which remedies may be most beneficial for their specific situations.

Lastly, while exploring herbal remedies and supplements, patients should not overlook the importance of a holistic approach to managing Parkinson's disease. Incorporating a balanced diet, regular exercise, and mental health support can complement any benefits derived from herbal and supplemental therapies. Community support groups can also provide valuable insights and shared experiences regarding alternative therapies. By staying informed, patients can navigate their journey with Parkinson's disease more effectively, ensuring they utilize all available resources for optimal health and well-being.

Evaluating the Effectiveness of Alternative Therapies

Evaluating the effectiveness of alternative therapies for Parkinson's disease involves a careful examination of various non-conventional treatment options that patients may consider alongside traditional medical approaches. These therapies can range from nutritional supplements and herbal remedies to more holistic practices such as acupuncture and mindfulness. It is crucial for patients to approach these alternatives with a critical mindset, ensuring that any chosen method is supported by credible research and fits well within their overall treatment plan. Understanding the potential benefits and limitations of these therapies can empower patients to make informed decisions.

One of the most common alternative therapies explored by Parkinson's patients is dietary modification. Nutrition plays a significant role in managing symptoms and improving overall health. Research suggests that certain diets, such as the Mediterranean diet, rich in fruits, vegetables, whole grains, and healthy fats, may offer protective benefits against neurodegeneration. Patients should evaluate how specific dietary changes affect their symptoms and consult with healthcare providers or nutritionists to tailor a plan that suits their individual needs.

Exercise is another vital component that is often integrated into alternative therapy regimens. Regular physical activity has shown promising results in enhancing mobility, balance, and overall quality of life for those with Parkinson's disease. Various forms of exercise, including tai chi, dance, and resistance training, can be beneficial. Patients are encouraged to assess which activities resonate with them and contribute positively to their physical and mental well-being. Engaging in community programs or group classes can also provide valuable social support, which is essential for emotional health.

Mindfulness and stress reduction techniques, such as meditation and yoga, are also gaining traction as alternative therapies. These practices can help manage anxiety and depression, which are common among Parkinson's patients. Evaluating the effectiveness of these methods often requires personal experimentation, as individuals may respond differently. Keeping a journal to track changes in mood, stress levels, and overall well-being can provide insight into what techniques are most beneficial.

Finally, it is essential for patients to remain vigilant about the credibility of any alternative therapy they consider. Engaging with healthcare professionals, reviewing scientific literature, and participating in support groups can provide invaluable guidance. Patients should prioritize therapies that complement conventional treatments rather than replace them, ensuring a well-rounded approach to managing Parkinson's disease. By carefully evaluating the effectiveness of alternative therapies, patients can enhance their quality of life and navigate the complexities of their condition with greater confidence.

Chapter 8: Assistive Technologies for Parkinson's Patients

Overview of Assistive Technologies

Assistive technologies encompass a range of devices and software designed to aid individuals in managing daily activities more effectively, especially for those living with Parkinson's Disease. These technologies can significantly enhance the quality of life for patients by addressing specific challenges associated with the disease, such as mobility issues, communication difficulties, and cognitive impairments. By integrating assistive technologies into their daily routines, patients can maintain greater independence and improve their overall well-being.

Mobility aids are among the most commonly used assistive technologies for Parkinson's patients. These devices include walkers, canes, and scooters that provide physical support and stability, helping individuals navigate their environment safely. In addition to traditional mobility aids, advanced options such as powered wheelchairs and customizable walking frames are increasingly available. These devices can be tailored to meet the unique needs of each patient, allowing for greater freedom and mobility while minimizing the risk of falls.

Communication technologies also play a crucial role in assisting patients with Parkinson's Disease. Many individuals experience speech difficulties, which can impact their ability to communicate effectively. Speech-generating devices, voice amplifiers, and smartphone applications designed to assist with communication can empower patients to express themselves more clearly. These technologies facilitate social interactions, reducing feelings of isolation and enhancing the overall quality of life for both patients and their caregivers.

Cognitive support tools are another essential category of assistive technologies. Patients with Parkinson's may encounter challenges related to memory, organization, and attention. Digital reminders, calendar applications, and task management software can help individuals stay organized and maintain their routines. These tools not only assist with daily tasks but also promote cognitive engagement, which is vital for maintaining mental health and emotional well-being.

As advancements in technology continue to evolve, the landscape of assistive devices for Parkinson's patients will expand. Innovations such as smart home systems, wearable health monitors, and telehealth services offer new opportunities for enhancing patient care. By staying informed about these developments, patients and caregivers can make better choices regarding their management strategies, ultimately leading to improved outcomes and a more fulfilling life despite the challenges presented by Parkinson's Disease.

Mobility Aids

Mobility aids play a crucial role in enhancing the quality of life for individuals diagnosed with Parkinson's disease. As the disease progresses, patients may experience a range of mobility challenges, including stiffness, tremors, and difficulties with balance. These impediments can significantly impact daily activities and overall independence. Understanding the various mobility aids available can empower patients and caregivers to make informed decisions about the tools that can best support mobility and safety.

One common mobility aid is the walker, which provides stability and support for those who may feel unsteady while walking. Walkers come in different designs, including standard walkers and those with wheels. The choice between these options often depends on the individual's strength and balance. For some, a rolling walker can facilitate smoother movement, allowing for a more natural gait. It is essential for patients to work with healthcare professionals to find the right fit and ensure that they are using the walker correctly to prevent falls and injuries.

Canes are another accessible option for those experiencing mild to moderate mobility issues. They can help redistribute weight and provide balance but may not be suitable for everyone. Patients should consider their specific needs and discuss them with their healthcare provider. The right cane can make a significant difference in day-to-day activities, allowing individuals to maintain a degree of independence while ensuring safety during ambulation.

In addition to traditional mobility aids, technology is also making strides in this area. Smart walking aids equipped with sensors can alert users to potential hazards, assist with navigation, and even monitor gait patterns. These advancements can provide valuable feedback and support, especially for those in the early stages of Parkinson's disease. Engaging with these technologies can help patients feel more secure when moving around, ultimately improving their confidence and willingness to engage in social activities.

Finally, it is essential to remember that mobility aids are not a one-size-fits-all solution. Individual preferences, lifestyle, and specific symptoms should guide the selection process. Working closely with occupational therapists and physiotherapists can help patients identify the most suitable aids for their unique circumstances. By exploring these options, individuals with Parkinson's disease can better navigate their environments, maintain their independence, and improve their overall well-being.

Communication Devices

Effective communication is essential for individuals living with Parkinson's disease, particularly as the condition progresses and may impact speech and language abilities. Various communication devices have emerged to assist patients in expressing their thoughts and needs more easily, thereby improving their quality of life. Understanding the options available can help patients and caregivers make informed choices about which devices might best suit their unique circumstances.

One of the most widely used communication devices is speech-generating devices (SGDs), which can convert text or symbols into spoken words. These devices range from simple applications on smartphones and tablets to sophisticated dedicated devices that offer a range of functions. Many SGDs allow users to customize their vocabulary and adjust speech output settings, enabling them to communicate in a way that feels most comfortable. Additionally, these devices can often be paired with other assistive technologies, such as eye-tracking systems, to further enhance communication for those who may have difficulty using their hands.

Another category of communication devices includes apps designed specifically for individuals with speech difficulties. These applications provide users with the ability to create phrases and sentences quickly. Some apps feature predictive text and symbol-based communication, allowing patients to convey complex thoughts without extensive typing. The convenience of using a smartphone or tablet makes these apps accessible and familiar for many patients, further supporting their independence in communication.

For those who may prefer or require more traditional methods, low-tech communication devices still play a significant role. These can include communication boards, picture cards, or symbol systems that allow for non-verbal communication. Caregivers and family members can work with patients to develop personalized boards that reflect their specific needs and preferences. This approach not only aids communication but also fosters a sense of agency for the patient, reinforcing their ability to engage actively with those around them.

Finally, it is important to recognize the role of community support groups in enhancing communication strategies. Many support groups offer resources and workshops focused on the use of communication devices, sharing experiences, and discussing best practices.

Engaging with others who face similar challenges can provide valuable insights and encouragement, helping patients feel less isolated in their journey. By combining the use of communication devices with community support, individuals with Parkinson's disease can better navigate the complexities of their condition and maintain meaningful connections with those around them.

Home Modifications and Smart Technology

Home modifications and the integration of smart technology can significantly enhance the quality of life for individuals living with Parkinson's disease. As the condition progresses, daily tasks can become increasingly challenging due to symptoms such as tremors, stiffness, and cognitive changes. By adapting the home environment, individuals can maintain independence and ensure safety. Simple modifications like removing rugs, installing grab bars in bathrooms, and ensuring adequate lighting can reduce the risk of falls and facilitate easier movement within the home.

Smart technology offers innovative solutions that can further assist in daily living. Devices such as voice-activated assistants can help manage tasks without the need for physical interaction, allowing patients to control lights, appliances, and even medical reminders through simple voice commands. For instance, a smart speaker can be programmed to provide medication alerts, ensuring that patients adhere to their treatment schedule. Additionally, smart home security systems can enhance safety by allowing caregivers to monitor the home environment remotely, providing peace of mind for both patients and their families.

The use of wearable technology is another area where smart devices can play a crucial role. Wearable fitness trackers, for example, can monitor physical activity levels and even track symptoms, providing valuable data that can be shared with healthcare providers. This information can help in tailoring exercise programs and adjusting treatment plans based on real-time feedback. Furthermore, some wearables are designed to detect falls, automatically alerting caregivers or emergency services if needed, thus offering an extra layer of security.

Assistive technologies, including mobility aids and communication devices, should also be considered in home modifications. Walkers, canes, and stairlifts can assist with mobility, while communication devices can help those experiencing speech difficulties. Investing in these tools can empower individuals to remain engaged in their daily routines and social interactions. Moreover, many of these technologies can be integrated with smart home systems, allowing for a seamless user experience that caters to specific needs.

Finally, it is essential for patients and caregivers to stay informed about the latest advancements in both home modifications and smart technology. Engaging with community support groups can provide valuable insights and resources tailored to managing Parkinson's disease. By embracing these modifications and technologies, individuals can create a supportive living environment that fosters independence, enhances safety, and ultimately improves their overall well-being.

Benefits of Technology in Daily Life

Technology has become an integral part of daily life, offering numerous benefits that can greatly enhance the lives of individuals with Parkinson's disease. From communication tools to health management apps, technology provides resources that can assist in managing symptoms, staying connected with caregivers, and accessing vital information. As patients navigate their journey with Parkinson's, leveraging these technological advancements can lead to improved quality of life and greater independence.

Assistive technologies play a crucial role in helping Parkinson's patients maintain their daily routines and manage their symptoms effectively. Devices such as smart home systems can facilitate easier control of the home environment, allowing individuals to adjust lighting, temperature, and security features with simple voice commands or mobile apps. This not only promotes safety but also encourages autonomy, enabling patients to remain in their homes longer and participate more actively in their daily lives.

Health management apps specifically designed for Parkinson's patients offer valuable features for tracking symptoms, medication schedules, and exercise routines. These tools can provide reminders for medication intake, monitor side effects, and even allow users to log their physical activity, which is essential for maintaining movement and flexibility. By utilizing these apps, patients can become proactive in their health management, fostering a sense of empowerment and control over their condition.

Technology also facilitates better communication between patients and caregivers. Telehealth services have emerged as a significant resource, allowing individuals to consult with healthcare providers remotely. This is particularly beneficial for those who may have difficulties traveling due to mobility issues. Regular virtual check-ups can ensure that patients receive timely advice and support, making it easier to adjust treatment plans and address concerns as they arise.

Moreover, online communities and support groups have flourished with the advent of social media and forums, providing patients and caregivers with a platform to connect, share experiences, and exchange valuable resources. These digital spaces can alleviate feelings of isolation and foster a sense of belonging among individuals navigating similar challenges. By embracing technology, Parkinson's patients can enhance their daily lives, improve their mental health, and build a supportive network that contributes to their overall well-being.

Chapter 9: Mental Health and Parkinson's Disease

Understanding the Mental Health Impact

Understanding the mental health impact of Parkinson's Disease is essential for patients and caregivers alike. Parkinson's not only affects physical mobility but also has profound psychological repercussions. Many patients experience a range of emotional challenges, including anxiety, depression, and feelings of isolation. Recognizing these symptoms early can significantly improve quality of life and lead to more effective management strategies. Awareness of mental health issues is crucial for patients to seek help and for caregivers to provide appropriate support.

The relationship between Parkinson's Disease and mental health can often be misunderstood. The neurological changes associated with Parkinson's can lead to alterations in mood and behavior, which may not solely stem from the stress of living with a chronic illness. For instance, the depletion of dopamine—a neurotransmitter that plays a key role in mood regulation—can contribute to feelings of sadness or apathy. Understanding this biological basis can help patients and caregivers recognize that these emotional challenges are not a personal failing but rather a consequence of the disease.

Moreover, the social stigma surrounding mental health can complicate these issues for Parkinson's patients. Many may feel hesitant to discuss their emotional struggles due to fear of judgment or misunderstanding from others. This silence can exacerbate feelings of loneliness and despair. Creating an open dialogue about mental health within the Parkinson's community is vital. Support groups offer a safe space for patients to share their experiences and feelings, fostering a sense of belonging and reducing isolation.

Incorporating mental health care into the overall treatment plan for Parkinson's Disease is essential. This can include therapy, medication, and lifestyle modifications such as nutrition and exercise, which have been shown to positively influence mental well-being. Engaging in regular physical activity not only helps with motor symptoms but can also improve mood and cognitive function. Nutrition plays a role as well; a balanced diet rich in antioxidants and omega-3 fatty acids may support brain health and enhance emotional resilience.

Lastly, ongoing research and advances in understanding the mental health implications of Parkinson's Disease continue to provide hope and new strategies for management. Innovative therapies, including cognitive behavioral therapy and mindfulness practices, are gaining traction as effective tools for improving mental health outcomes. As the field evolves, staying informed about these advances can empower patients and caregivers to make proactive choices regarding their mental health care. Recognizing the importance of mental health is not only a critical aspect of managing Parkinson's but also a step toward achieving a more fulfilling life despite the challenges of the disease.

Common Mental Health Issues

Common mental health issues associated with Parkinson's disease can significantly impact the quality of life for patients. Depression is one of the most prevalent mental health challenges faced by individuals with Parkinson's. Studies suggest that nearly 40% of Parkinson's patients experience depression at some point during their illness. This condition may stem from a combination of biological factors related to the disease, such as changes in brain chemistry, as well as emotional responses to the diagnosis and its progression. Recognizing the signs of depression, such as persistent sadness, fatigue, and loss of interest in previously enjoyed activities, is crucial for timely intervention and support.

Anxiety is another common mental health issue that often accompanies Parkinson's disease. Patients may experience a range of anxiety disorders, including generalized anxiety disorder, panic disorder, and social anxiety. The unpredictability of motor symptoms, coupled with concerns about future health and independence, can exacerbate feelings of anxiety. Symptoms such as restlessness, rapid heartbeat, and excessive worry can interfere with daily life and exacerbate other Parkinson's symptoms. Understanding these mental health challenges is vital for patients and caregivers, as effective management of anxiety can lead to improved overall well-being.

Cognitive impairment is also a significant concern for those living with Parkinson's disease. While it is often associated with the later stages of the condition, early cognitive changes can occur and may manifest as difficulty concentrating, memory problems, and challenges with decision-making. These cognitive symptoms can impact the ability to follow treatment plans, engage in social activities, and maintain independence. Patients and caregivers should be aware of these changes and communicate with healthcare providers to develop strategies that support cognitive health and enhance daily functioning.

Sleep disturbances are frequently reported among Parkinson's patients, contributing to the overall mental health burden. Insomnia, restless leg syndrome, and excessive daytime sleepiness can complicate the management of Parkinson's disease. Poor sleep quality not only affects mood and cognitive function but can also exacerbate motor symptoms. Addressing sleep issues through lifestyle changes, proper sleep hygiene, and potential interventions can help improve mental health outcomes and overall quality of life for patients.

Finally, the intersection of mental health and Parkinson's disease emphasizes the importance of community support and resources. Engaging with support groups, both for patients and caregivers, can provide a platform for sharing experiences and coping strategies. Mental health professionals specializing in Parkinson's can offer tailored interventions, including therapy and medication when necessary. By fostering an environment of understanding and support, patients can better navigate the complexities of mental health challenges associated with Parkinson's disease, ultimately leading to a more fulfilling life amidst the challenges posed by their condition.

Strategies for Maintaining Mental Well-Being

Maintaining mental well-being is crucial for individuals living with Parkinson's disease, especially in the early stages when symptoms may begin to emerge. One effective strategy is the incorporation of a structured daily routine. Establishing a predictable schedule can foster a sense of control and stability, which is often challenged by the unpredictable nature of Parkinson's. This routine should include time for activities that promote both mental and physical health, such as engaging hobbies, social interactions, and regular exercise. By prioritizing these activities, patients can create a balanced lifestyle that supports both their physical and emotional needs.

Engagement in social activities plays a significant role in mental health for those with Parkinson's. Isolation can exacerbate feelings of anxiety and depression, making it essential to stay connected with friends, family, and support groups. Participating in community support groups specifically for Parkinson's patients offers the opportunity to share experiences and coping strategies, which can alleviate feelings of loneliness. Additionally, social interactions provide emotional support and encourage individuals to express their feelings in a safe environment, fostering a sense of belonging and understanding.

Exercise is another vital component of mental well-being. Research has shown that physical activity can significantly improve mood and cognitive function in Parkinson's patients. Activities such as walking, swimming, or engaging in yoga can not only enhance physical health but also boost endorphin levels, which are known to elevate mood. Furthermore, group exercise classes designed for individuals with Parkinson's can combine the benefits of physical activity with social interaction, reinforcing both physical and mental resilience.

Nutrition also plays an essential role in maintaining mental health. A balanced diet rich in antioxidants, omega-3 fatty acids, and vitamins can support brain health and improve mood stability. Patients should consider incorporating foods such as leafy greens, fatty fish, nuts, and whole grains into their diets. Staying hydrated and managing caffeine and sugar intake can also contribute to better mental clarity and emotional regulation. Consulting with a nutritionist who specializes in Parkinson's can provide tailored dietary strategies that align with individual health needs.

Finally, mindfulness and relaxation techniques can serve as powerful tools for managing stress and enhancing mental well-being. Practices such as meditation, deep breathing exercises, and mindfulness can help patients cultivate a greater awareness of their thoughts and feelings, allowing for more effective coping strategies. These techniques can reduce anxiety and improve overall quality of life. By integrating mindfulness into their daily routines, patients can develop a more positive outlook, enabling them to navigate the challenges of Parkinson's disease with greater resilience and peace of mind.

Seeking Professional Help

Seeking professional help is a crucial step in managing Parkinson's disease, particularly during its early stages. Recognizing the initial symptoms can be overwhelming, and understanding when to consult a healthcare provider is essential. Early intervention can lead to more effective treatment plans and better management of symptoms. It is vital to reach out to neurologists who specialize in movement disorders, as they possess the expertise necessary to diagnose and recommend appropriate therapies tailored to individual needs.

During your visit to a healthcare professional, it is important to discuss all symptoms, no matter how minor they may seem. Early signs of Parkinson's disease, such as tremors, rigidity, or changes in coordination, should be openly communicated. Additionally, patients should consider keeping a diary of symptoms to provide the doctor with a comprehensive view of their experiences. This information can help the professional in making an accurate diagnosis and in determining the most suitable treatment options available.

Aside from neurologists, other healthcare professionals, including physical therapists, occupational therapists, and nutritionists, can play a significant role in the management of Parkinson's disease. A physical therapist can develop an exercise regimen that enhances mobility and strength, while an occupational therapist can assist in adapting daily activities to maintain independence. Nutritionists can provide guidance on dietary adjustments that might alleviate some symptoms and improve overall health. Collaborating with a team of specialists can create a holistic approach to managing the disease.

Support for mental health is another critical aspect of seeking professional help. Many individuals with Parkinson's experience anxiety, depression, or mood swings, which can significantly impact their quality of life. Consulting with mental health professionals who understand the psychological aspects of chronic illnesses can be beneficial. They can offer therapeutic interventions and coping strategies to help navigate the emotional challenges associated with Parkinson's disease.

Finally, community support groups can provide invaluable resources and connections for both patients and caregivers. Engaging with others who are experiencing similar challenges can foster a sense of belonging and understanding. These groups often invite healthcare professionals to speak about the latest advances in research, treatment options, and alternative therapies. Building a strong support network not only enhances the management of Parkinson's disease but also empowers patients and their families to face the journey with resilience and hope.

Support Systems for Mental Health

Support systems for mental health play a crucial role in managing the emotional and psychological challenges associated with

Parkinson's Disease. Patients may experience a range of mental health issues, including anxiety, depression, and cognitive changes, which can significantly affect their quality of life. Recognizing the importance of mental health is essential for both patients and caregivers, as these issues can exacerbate physical symptoms and hinder overall well-being. It is vital to establish a robust support network that encompasses both professional and community resources tailored to the unique needs of individuals with Parkinson's.

Professional mental health support typically includes therapy, counseling, and psychiatric services. Psychologists and counselors can help patients navigate their feelings, develop coping strategies, and address specific concerns related to Parkinson's. Cognitive Behavioral Therapy (CBT) has shown particular promise in helping manage anxiety and depression among patients. Additionally, psychiatrists may recommend medications to alleviate severe symptoms. It is beneficial for patients to work closely with their healthcare team to create a treatment plan that integrates mental health care with their overall Parkinson's management strategy.

Community support groups are another vital element of a comprehensive mental health support system. These groups provide a platform for patients to share their experiences, challenges, and triumphs with others who understand their journey. Engaging with peers can foster a sense of belonging and reduce feelings of isolation, which are common among those living with chronic conditions. Many organizations dedicated to Parkinson's Disease offer regular meetings, workshops, and activities designed to promote social interaction and emotional support, empowering patients and caregivers alike.

Family and caregiver support is equally important in the mental health landscape for Parkinson's patients. Caregivers often face their own mental health challenges, as they balance the demands of caregiving with their personal lives. Providing caregivers with access to resources, such as respite care, counseling, and education on Parkinson's, can alleviate stress and improve their ability to support their loved ones. Open communication between patients and caregivers about mental health needs can strengthen their relationship, ensuring that both parties feel heard and supported.

Incorporating wellness practices into daily routines can also enhance mental health for those with Parkinson's. Regular physical activity, a balanced diet, and mindfulness practices such as meditation or yoga can contribute to overall mental well-being. These activities not only improve physical health but also promote emotional resilience. Patients are encouraged to explore various avenues of support, including alternative therapies, and to remain proactive in seeking resources that address both their mental and physical health needs. By fostering a comprehensive support system, individuals can better navigate the complexities of Parkinson's Disease and enhance their quality of life.

Chapter 10: Community Support Groups for Parkinson's

Importance of Community Support

Community support plays a crucial role in the lives of individuals diagnosed with Parkinson's disease. It encompasses not only emotional assistance but also practical resources that can help patients navigate the complexities of their condition. Engaging with a supportive community allows patients to share experiences, seek advice, and find solace in knowing they are not alone in their journey. This network can include family, friends, healthcare providers, and trained support groups specifically focused on the needs of those living with Parkinson's.

The emotional aspect of living with Parkinson's can be overwhelming. Feelings of isolation and anxiety are common, particularly in the early stages when symptoms begin to manifest. Community support groups provide a safe space for patients to express their fears and concerns. These gatherings foster an environment of understanding and empathy, where individuals can connect with others facing similar challenges. Sharing stories and coping strategies can empower patients, helping them to feel more in control of their lives and less burdened by their diagnosis.

In addition to emotional support, community networks can offer practical resources that are invaluable for managing Parkinson's disease. These resources may include information about local healthcare services, access to physical therapy, and nutritional guidance tailored to the unique needs of Parkinson's patients. Community members often share recommendations for assistive technologies that can enhance mobility and independence, making daily tasks more manageable. By pooling knowledge and experiences, the community can provide a wealth of information that can significantly improve the quality of life for patients.

Moreover, community support is essential for caregivers, who often experience their own set of challenges. Caregivers play a vital role in the daily lives of Parkinson's patients, and their emotional and physical well-being is equally important. Support groups for caregivers can offer respite, allowing them to share their experiences and learn from one another. These groups can provide resources for self-care, stress management, and coping strategies, ensuring that caregivers remain healthy and capable of providing the necessary support to their loved ones.

Finally, as research continues to advance in the field of Parkinson's disease, community support can serve as a bridge between new findings and patient awareness. Community organizations often host educational events, bringing in healthcare professionals to discuss the latest research, treatment options, and alternative therapies. Staying informed about advances in the understanding of Parkinson's can empower patients and caregivers to make educated decisions about their care. Ultimately, the importance of community support cannot be overstated; it is a foundation upon which patients and their families can build resilience, hope, and a better quality of life as they navigate the challenges of Parkinson's disease.

Types of Support Groups

Support groups play a crucial role in the lives of individuals affected by Parkinson's disease, providing an environment where patients, caregivers, and families can share experiences, gain insights, and find solace in community. There are various types of support groups catering to the unique needs of different individuals in the Parkinson's community. These groups may be organized by specific demographics, stages of the disease, or shared interests, making it essential for participants to identify which type best suits their circumstances and preferences.

One common type of support group focuses on early-stage Parkinson's patients. These groups often emphasize awareness and education regarding early symptoms, allowing members to discuss their experiences and challenges while navigating the initial stages of the disease. Participants can exchange valuable information about recognizing symptoms, coping mechanisms, and lifestyle changes, such as nutrition and diet adjustments tailored for early-stage patients. This supportive environment fosters empowerment and encourages proactive management of health and well-being.

Support groups may also be tailored specifically for caregivers, who often face their own set of challenges while supporting a loved one with Parkinson's. Caregiver support groups provide a safe space for sharing feelings, frustrations, and strategies for coping with the demands of caregiving. These groups can offer practical resources on self-care, mental health, and effective communication with healthcare providers, ensuring that caregivers are not only equipped to support their loved ones but also prioritize their own well-being.

Another type of support group centers around physical health and exercise, recognizing the importance of movement therapy in managing Parkinson's symptoms. These groups might incorporate physical activities, such as yoga or tai chi, alongside discussions about physical therapy techniques and the benefits of maintaining an active lifestyle. Participants can share their personal experiences related to exercise routines, nutritional advice, and advancements in research that highlight the importance of staying active in managing Parkinson's disease effectively.

Finally, online support groups have become increasingly popular, especially for those who may have difficulty attending in-person meetings due to mobility issues or geographic constraints. These virtual platforms allow individuals to connect with a broader community, sharing experiences and resources without the limitations of physical distance. Online groups can encompass a wide range of topics, from alternative therapies and assistive technologies to mental health resources, providing flexibility and accessibility for all members of the Parkinson's community.

How to Find a Support Group

Finding a support group can be a crucial step for individuals navigating the early signs of Parkinson's Disease. These groups provide an invaluable platform where patients and caregivers can share experiences, gain insights, and receive emotional support. To begin your search, consider local hospitals or clinics that specialize in neurology. Many medical facilities host support groups or can connect you with organizations that do. Additionally, reaching out to your healthcare provider can yield recommendations tailored specifically to your needs, ensuring that you find a group that resonates with your situation.

Online resources have become increasingly popular for those seeking support. Websites dedicated to Parkinson's Disease often feature directories of local and virtual support groups. Organizations such as the Parkinson's Foundation and the Michael J. Fox Foundation offer comprehensive listings that can help you find groups based on your geographic location or specific interests, such as diet, exercise, or caregiver support. Engaging with these online platforms can also facilitate connections with fellow patients, providing a sense of community that transcends geographical barriers.

Social media is another powerful tool for connecting with support groups. Platforms like Facebook have numerous groups dedicated to Parkinson's Disease, where members share personal stories, tips for symptom management, and resources for caregivers. These digital communities can foster a sense of belonging and provide immediate access to information and support. However, it's vital to approach these groups with an open mind while critically evaluating the information shared, as the quality of advice can vary.

When considering joining a support group, it's essential to evaluate the group's focus and dynamics. Some groups may concentrate on specific aspects of living with Parkinson's, such as mental health or alternative therapies, while others might offer a more general approach. Attend a few meetings or sessions to see if the group feels like a good fit. Pay attention to the level of openness and support among members, as a welcoming environment can significantly enhance your experience and comfort level in sharing your journey.

Finally, don't hesitate to create your own support system if existing groups do not meet your needs. This could involve gathering a few friends or family members to discuss your experiences and challenges, or even starting a new group that focuses on a specific niche, such as nutrition for Parkinson's patients. Community building is essential, and by taking the initiative, you can cultivate a supportive network that addresses your unique situation and fosters resilience in the face of Parkinson's Disease.

Benefits of Peer Support

Peer support offers numerous benefits for individuals navigating the early signs of Parkinson's Disease. For patients, connecting with others who share similar experiences can significantly reduce feelings of isolation and loneliness. Engaging with peers allows individuals to discuss their challenges openly, fostering an environment of empathy and understanding. This connection can enhance emotional well-being, as patients often feel validated by others who truly understand their struggles and triumphs.

One of the key advantages of peer support is the exchange of practical advice and coping strategies. Patients can share insights about managing early symptoms, such as tremors or fatigue, and discuss effective ways to incorporate nutrition and exercise into their daily routines. This collaborative approach not only empowers individuals to take control of their health but also encourages them to stay proactive in their treatment journey. Learning from the experiences of others can lead to discovering new resources or therapies that might have otherwise gone unnoticed.

Peer support also plays a vital role in mental health. The emotional toll of a Parkinson's diagnosis can be substantial, often leading to feelings of anxiety and depression. Participating in support groups or connecting with peers can provide a safe space for expressing these emotions and finding reassurance. Members can share their fears and successes, helping to cultivate a sense of hope and resilience. This collective support can be instrumental in promoting a positive mindset and reinforcing the importance of mental health care alongside physical treatment.

In addition to emotional and practical benefits, peer support can enhance access to valuable resources. Many support groups offer information on the latest advances in Parkinson's research, alternative therapies, and assistive technologies that can improve daily living. Patients who participate in these networks often find themselves more informed and better equipped to navigate their healthcare options. Furthermore, caregivers can benefit from these interactions, gaining insights from others who face similar challenges in providing support.

Ultimately, the benefits of peer support extend beyond individual experiences and contribute to a stronger community. Building relationships with others affected by Parkinson's fosters a sense of solidarity and collective strength. As individuals share their journeys, they create a network of support that can advocate for awareness and resources within the broader community. This united front not only uplifts those directly affected by Parkinson's but also promotes greater understanding and support from society at large.

Building a Support Network

Building a support network is essential for individuals navigating the early signs of Parkinson's Disease. Establishing a robust support system can significantly enhance emotional well-being, provide practical assistance, and foster a sense of community. This network can include family, friends, healthcare professionals, and support groups specifically tailored for Parkinson's patients. Each component of this network plays a vital role in helping individuals manage their symptoms, share experiences, and gain access to valuable resources.

Family and friends are often the first line of support for someone facing a diagnosis of Parkinson's Disease. Open communication is crucial, as it allows loved ones to understand the challenges faced by the patient. Encouraging family members to participate in educational sessions or workshops on Parkinson's can empower them to provide informed support. Additionally, sharing information about early symptoms and coping strategies can help alleviate feelings of isolation and confusion, fostering a more supportive home environment.

Healthcare professionals are another critical component of a support network. Building strong relationships with neurologists, physical therapists, nutritionists, and mental health providers can ensure a comprehensive approach to managing the disease. Regular appointments and open dialogue with these professionals can provide patients with tailored treatment plans, dietary recommendations, and exercise regimens that are essential for maintaining health. A multidisciplinary team can address various aspects of the disease, allowing patients to receive holistic care that caters to their unique needs.

Community support groups offer an invaluable resource for those living with Parkinson's Disease. These groups create a safe space for patients to share their experiences, fears, and triumphs, fostering a sense of belonging. Connecting with others who face similar challenges can help individuals recognize that they are not alone in their journey. Many support groups also provide access to educational resources, guest speakers, and workshops on topics ranging from mental health to exercise and nutrition, enriching the patient's understanding of their condition.

Lastly, exploring online resources and virtual support communities can broaden the network even further. Websites dedicated to Parkinson's Disease often feature forums, webinars, and articles that can educate and inspire patients. Social media platforms can also connect individuals with similar experiences, allowing for the exchange of tips, encouragement, and friendship. By actively building a diverse support network, patients can better navigate the complexities of Parkinson's Disease, enhancing their quality of life and resilience in the face of challenges.

Chapter 11: Genetic Factors in Parkinson's Disease

Overview of Genetic Research

Genetic research has become a pivotal area of study in understanding Parkinson's Disease (PD). As scientists delve deeper into the genetic underpinnings of this neurodegenerative disorder, they are uncovering the complex interactions between inherited traits and environmental factors that may contribute to the onset of symptoms. While the majority of Parkinson's cases are classified as sporadic, meaning they occur without a clear familial link, a subset of patients exhibits hereditary forms of the disease. Identifying these genetic markers not only aids in early diagnosis but also opens the door to potential targeted therapies tailored to individual genetic profiles.

The most significant genetic contributions to Parkinson's Disease have been linked to mutations in specific genes, such as SNCA, LRRK2, and PARK7. The SNCA gene encodes alpha-synuclein, a protein that plays a crucial role in synaptic function and is implicated in the formation of Lewy bodies, hallmark features of PD. Mutations in the LRRK2 gene are the most common genetic cause of familial Parkinson's and have also been associated with sporadic cases. Understanding these genetic factors allows researchers to explore how they influence the disease's progression and symptoms, paving the way for novel therapeutic interventions.

Recent advancements in genetic research techniques, including whole-genome sequencing and genome-wide association studies (GWAS), have accelerated the discovery of additional risk factors for Parkinson's. These techniques enable scientists to analyze large datasets, identifying genetic variations that may predispose individuals to the disease. Moreover, the integration of bioinformatics tools helps in interpreting complex genetic data, allowing for a more comprehensive understanding of how various genes interact and contribute to the pathology of Parkinson's. As these technologies continue to evolve, they promise to enhance our knowledge of genetic predisposition and its implications for disease management.

The implications of genetic research extend beyond understanding the disease; they also hold significant promise for personalized medicine. By identifying specific genetic mutations, healthcare providers can develop tailored treatment plans that consider a patient's unique genetic makeup. This personalized approach may improve treatment efficacy and minimize adverse effects, ultimately enhancing the quality of life for individuals living with Parkinson's. Furthermore, genetic counseling can provide patients and their families with valuable information regarding the hereditary nature of the disease, empowering them to make informed decisions about their health and care.

As genetic research continues to advance, it is essential for Parkinson's patients and caregivers to stay informed about emerging findings and their potential impact on treatment strategies. Engaging with healthcare professionals about genetic testing and its implications can help patients navigate their options, leading to more effective management of the disease. Additionally, participating in community support groups and educational resources can foster a better understanding of genetic factors in Parkinson's, promoting awareness and advocacy within the broader Parkinson's community. This collective effort not only enhances individual patient care but also contributes to the ongoing research efforts aimed at unraveling the complexities of Parkinson's Disease.

Identifying Genetic Risk Factors

Identifying genetic risk factors is a crucial step in understanding the potential development of Parkinson's Disease (PD). Research indicates that certain genetic mutations can increase an individual's susceptibility to Parkinson's, making it essential for patients and caregivers to be aware of these factors. While the majority of PD cases are sporadic, approximately 10 to 15 percent are familial, meaning they occur in families and can often be traced to specific genetic mutations. The most well-known among these mutations are found in the SNCA, LRRK2, PARK7, PINK1, and PRKN genes. Recognizing these genetic connections can help in early detection and management of the disease.

Genetic testing has become an increasingly important tool in identifying those at risk for Parkinson's Disease. For individuals with a family history of PD, consulting with a genetic counselor may provide insights into whether genetic testing is appropriate. This process involves analyzing DNA to find mutations associated with an increased risk of developing the disease. For patients who test positive for these mutations, it can lead to more proactive monitoring for early symptoms, potentially facilitating earlier interventions that may slow disease progression.

Understanding the implications of genetic risk factors also extends beyond testing. Knowledge of genetic predispositions can empower patients and their families to make informed lifestyle choices that may mitigate some risks associated with Parkinson's. Research has shown that factors such as diet, exercise, and social engagement can play a role in overall brain health. For example, a diet rich in antioxidants, omega-3 fatty acids, and vitamins may help support neurological function, while regular physical activity can improve mobility and reduce the severity of symptoms.

Moreover, the identification of genetic risk factors can foster a greater sense of community among patients and caregivers. By sharing experiences related to genetic predispositions, individuals can find support and understanding in shared challenges. Community support groups offer a platform for discussing not only the emotional aspects of living with PD but also practical strategies for coping with the genetic aspects of the disease. Connecting with others who have similar experiences can alleviate feelings of isolation and provide valuable resources for navigating the complexities of Parkinson's.

As research continues to advance, the understanding of genetic factors in Parkinson's Disease is likely to evolve. This ongoing research may lead to the development of targeted therapies aimed at specific genetic mutations, potentially transforming the landscape of PD treatment. Staying informed about the latest advancements in genetic research can empower patients and caregivers alike, providing hope for future interventions that could significantly improve quality of life for those affected by this challenging condition.

Genetic Testing and Counseling

Genetic testing and counseling play a pivotal role in understanding the complexities of Parkinson's disease, particularly for individuals who may be at risk due to family history or genetic predispositions. As research advances, it becomes increasingly clear that certain genetic factors can influence the likelihood of developing Parkinson's disease. Genetic testing can identify mutations associated with the condition, such as those in the SNCA, LRRK2, and PARK7 genes. For patients and their families, knowing whether they carry these mutations can provide valuable information for making informed decisions about health management and lifestyle choices.

Counseling is an essential component of the genetic testing process. It offers patients and their families the opportunity to discuss the implications of test results in a supportive environment. A genetic counselor can help clarify the uncertainties surrounding genetic risk, explain the inheritance patterns, and address any emotional concerns that may arise from the testing process. This support is crucial, as learning about potential genetic risks can lead to anxiety or fear about the future. Counselors help navigate these feelings and provide resources for coping and planning.

Understanding genetic risks can also assist in early detection and intervention strategies. If a genetic predisposition to Parkinson's disease is identified, patients may choose to engage in preventative measures, such as lifestyle modifications, dietary changes, and regular exercise, which are known to contribute positively to overall health. Early engagement with healthcare providers can facilitate monitoring for early symptoms and possibly lead to earlier treatment, which may improve quality of life and potentially slow disease progression.

Moreover, genetic testing can enhance the personalization of treatment approaches. As research continues to uncover the interplay between genetics and the efficacy of various therapies, healthcare providers can tailor treatment plans based on an individual's genetic makeup. This might include pharmacogenomics, where medications are prescribed based on how a patient's genetic profile affects their response to certain drugs. Such personalized strategies can lead to more effective management of symptoms and a better overall experience for patients living with Parkinson's disease.

Finally, it is essential to foster a community that supports individuals navigating the complexities of genetic testing and counseling. Support groups and online forums can provide a platform for patients and their families to share experiences, seek advice, and connect with others who understand their journey. Access to community resources can alleviate feelings of isolation and empower individuals with knowledge and support as they navigate the implications of genetic testing in relation to Parkinson's disease. By fostering open discussions about genetic risks, patients can better understand their health and advocate for their needs within the healthcare system.

Implications for Patients and Families

Understanding the early signs of Parkinson's Disease is crucial for patients and their families, as it enables timely intervention and management strategies that can significantly improve quality of life. Early recognition of symptoms such as tremors, rigidity, and changes in balance allows for proactive measures to be implemented. Patients can benefit from establishing a comprehensive care plan that includes regular consultations with healthcare providers, ensuring that both medical and lifestyle factors are addressed. This collaborative approach fosters an environment where patients feel empowered to take control of their health journey.

For families, being educated about Parkinson's Disease is equally important. Family members often play a critical role in supporting patients through their experiences with the disease. By understanding the implications of early symptoms, families can better assist their loved ones in navigating daily challenges. This support can range from helping with mobility issues to encouraging adherence to prescribed therapies, including physical exercise and proper nutrition. Knowledge of the disease equips families to make informed decisions and advocate effectively for the needs of their loved ones.

Nutrition and diet are essential components of managing Parkinson's symptoms. Patients and families should focus on a balanced diet rich in antioxidants, omega-3 fatty acids, and other nutrients that can support brain health and overall well-being. It is beneficial to consult with a nutritionist familiar with Parkinson's to create personalized meal plans that cater to individual needs and preferences. Educating families about the significance of nutrition helps them to encourage and prepare healthy meals, creating a supportive home environment that directly contributes to the patient's health.

Exercise and physical therapy play a pivotal role in maintaining mobility and reducing the progression of symptoms. Families can encourage patients to engage in regular physical activities tailored to their abilities. Support groups and community resources can provide valuable information on local exercise programs designed specifically for individuals with Parkinson's. By participating in these activities together, families can foster a sense of community and motivation, reinforcing the importance of physical well-being in managing the disease.

Finally, mental health considerations are integral to the overall care of Parkinson's patients. The emotional impact of a Parkinson's diagnosis can be profound, affecting both patients and their families. It is vital to seek mental health support, whether through counseling or support groups, to address feelings of anxiety, depression, or isolation that may arise. Families should be encouraged to engage in open conversations about mental health, facilitating a supportive atmosphere where patients feel comfortable sharing their feelings and experiences. This holistic approach to care not only enhances the quality of life for patients but also strengthens familial bonds as they navigate the challenges of Parkinson's Disease together.

Future Directions in Genetic Research

Future directions in genetic research hold significant promise for understanding and managing Parkinson's Disease. As scientists delve deeper into the genetic underpinnings of this complex condition, new insights are emerging that could lead to earlier diagnosis, more personalized treatment strategies, and potentially even preventive measures. The exploration of genetic factors associated with Parkinson's not only enhances our understanding of the disease but also opens the door to innovative approaches that may improve the quality of life for patients and their caregivers.

Recent advancements in genomic technologies, such as whole-genome sequencing and CRISPR gene editing, have made it easier to identify genetic variants linked to Parkinson's Disease. Researchers are increasingly focusing on genes known to be associated with familial forms of Parkinson's, such as SNCA, LRRK2, and PARK7. Understanding how these genetic mutations influence the onset and progression of the disease could lead to targeted therapies that address the root causes rather than merely alleviating symptoms. As the field progresses, we may see the development of genetic tests that can predict the likelihood of developing Parkinson's, allowing for proactive management and lifestyle changes.

In addition to identifying genetic markers, future research will likely emphasize the interaction between genetics and environmental factors. It is becoming increasingly clear that genetics alone does not determine the course of Parkinson's Disease. Factors such as diet, physical activity, and exposure to toxins play a crucial role in how the disease manifests. By studying these interactions, researchers aim to create comprehensive models that better reflect the multifaceted nature of Parkinson's, helping patients and caregivers make informed choices about lifestyle interventions that could mitigate symptoms or delay progression.

Another promising direction in genetic research is the exploration of gene therapy as a potential treatment. Early-stage clinical trials are investigating the feasibility of delivering therapeutic genes directly to the brain, aiming to restore normal function or protect neurons from degeneration. If successful, these approaches could revolutionize the way Parkinson's is treated, shifting the focus from symptomatic relief to addressing the underlying biological processes. The development of advanced delivery systems, such as viral vectors, is crucial for ensuring that these therapies can effectively reach the targeted areas in the brain.

As genetic research continues to advance, it is essential to integrate these findings into practical applications that benefit patients and their families. Education and awareness about genetic factors in Parkinson's Disease can empower patients to engage in discussions with their healthcare providers about genetic testing and personalized treatment options. Furthermore, as research uncovers more about the genetic landscape of Parkinson's, community support groups can play a vital role in disseminating information, fostering connections, and providing resources that help individuals navigate their journey with Parkinson's. The future of genetic research in Parkinson's is bright, promising a deeper understanding of the disease and paving the way for enhanced care and support for those affected.